CONQUER YOUR CRAVINGS

Four Steps to Stopping the Struggle and
Winning Your Inner Battle with Food

Second Edition

By

Suzanne Giesemann

Aventine Press

Also by Suzanne Giesemann:

The Priest and the Medium: *The Amazing True Story of Psychic Medium B. Anne Gehman and Her Husband, Former Jesuit Priest Wayne Knoll, Ph.D*

It's Your Boat Too:
A Woman's Guide to Greater Enjoyment on the Water

Living a Dream: *A Journey from Aide to the Chairman of the Joint Chiefs of Staff on 9/11 to Full-Time Cruiser*

To Ty

Published by Aventine Press
750 State St. #319
San Diego CA, 92101

www.aventinepress.com

Cover design by Rob Johnson, www.johnsondesign.org
Author photo by Eric Smith, Captured Moments Photography

ISBN: 1-59330-606-7
Printed in the United States of America

Contents

Preface

This is not a diet book. I'm not going to tell you how to lose ten pounds in ten days and I won't be recommending a new way to exercise without breaking a sweat.

What I will offer you, however, is something much more satisfying. I'll offer you peace of mind, freedom from obsession with food, and an end to the constant struggle with the question: to eat or not to eat?

I'll also offer change—change in the way you think about food and change in the way you react to it.

Rather than telling you what foods to eliminate from your diet, I'll give you food for thought. I'll show you a step-by-step process to follow when you're confronted with the unwanted urge to eat. You'll learn how to use this process to root out nonproductive thoughts and behaviors and to be more aware of why you act the way you do around food. You'll have the chance to practice successful techniques for dealing with your cravings that will produce immediate results.

So what makes me an expert on conquering cravings?

Do I have a degree in nutrition? No, but like anyone who's ever obsessed about food, I can tell you exactly how many calories are in a slice of bread or how many grams of fat are in a Hershey bar. Do I have a Ph.D. in psychology? No, but my bookshelves used to be lined with enough self-help books to start a library. Have I lost a hundred pounds? No, I can't make that claim either. But as you'll soon learn, a person doesn't have to be overweight to have a problem with food.

You may be carrying around a few extra pounds, but you could just as easily have the body of a supermodel and still be miserable because of the way you deal with food. Many people who appear healthy and happy on the outside are caught in an inner battle with food, constantly struggling with cravings which compel them to eat, even when they don't want to.

So why am I qualified to write a book about overcoming cravings? When it comes to obsessing about food, I can honestly say, "Been there, done that."

From the time I was a teenager sneaking cookies or ice cream to try to quiet nearly constant cravings, until well into my adult years when I couldn't concentrate on work until I'd eaten a candy bar or two, food was my major fixation. For more than eighteen years I felt I was under its power. I felt I was controlled by my cravings. They kept me from fully enjoying the people and things around me, and they made me miserable.

But more important than having been there is the reason I'm writing this book now: *I'm not there anymore.*

Cravings no longer rule my life, but it wasn't easy getting to this point. Countless books, motivational tapes, and self-therapy sessions led me stumbling down a trail of trial and error until I finally forged the kind of healthy relationship with food I'd always thought was beyond my reach.

The long and difficult road to finding my cure is what led me to write this book. I wanted to pull together the things that had worked for me that I'd been unable to find in any one place and make it easier for others who are still struggling. The peace of mind I feel at being free from those ever-present, self destructive cravings is what compels me to share the keys to my cure in one compact reference for those who are still under food's false spell.

I know the process that worked for me will work for you. It will work for *anyone* who is preoccupied with food and eating because it attacks the problems universal to all cravers. Any *one* of the strategies in the process you are about to learn can be used to stop a craving in an instant. When packaged together in this easy-to-remember four-step process, they create a virtual arsenal of ammunition you can use to conquer your cravings once and for all.

I've recovered from compulsive overeating. Yes, I still get occasional cravings, but I no longer react to them with fear. I've learned how to deal with them in a healthy way. I was extremely fortunate that my preoccupation with food never progressed to the stage where my actions harmed me physically. I never reached the dangerous extremes of the eating disorder spectrum, bounded by anorexia nervosa at one end and bulimia at the other.

This book focuses, therefore, on the middle ground. It's intended for those whose cravings are interfering with their happiness, but whose preoccupation with food has not led to self-destructive behaviors. Appendix A lists some of the signs of a person with a serious eating disorder. If you recognize yourself in these descriptions, I strongly urge you to seek the help of a professional trained in this field. While anorexics or bulimics can benefit from the strategies in this book, they may be better served by getting one-on-one personal support. Because I don't have counseling credentials or a psychology degree, in the course of writing this book I sometimes doubted I had the proper qualifications to be giving advice to others. Fortunately, one day when I was wrestling with a bad case of writer's block, I struck up a conversation with a woman in the waiting room of my doctor's office. She'd been browsing through a magazine and commented on an article she'd just read about a new diet program. We chatted for a while about food and women's preoccupation with weight. Eventually we got around to the fact that I was writing a book about overcoming cravings, and I mentioned I was having some trouble. I was surprised when she showed more than casual interest in my efforts.

Here was a woman who appeared totally content with herself, but she suddenly stared down at the floor and admitted that food cravings were a big problem for her. After a moment she looked up and said, "Don't stop writing. This is one of those things people who have never suffered with will never understand. The ones who truly know how to defeat something are those who've faced it."

I have faced it, and I'm confident that the techniques and ideas you'll learn from this book will help you defeat your cravings once and for all. I must warn you, however, that if you've been fighting cravings for years, they won't magically disappear when you finish the final chapter. It will take dedicated effort to rid yourself of years of incorrect thinking and self-defeating behaviors.

If you diligently apply the techniques in this book, however, I can promise you small victories right from the start. Each time you work through a craving without giving in you'll be able to chalk up yet another accomplishment to add to your list of successes. These small victories will build upon themselves until gradually you'll notice fewer and fewer cravings. You won't panic when they hit because you will have overcome them in the past and you'll know what to do to get through them again.

If you're willing to commit yourself to overcoming your preoccupation with food, I know you'll be successful. Getting there will be an adventure in itself, as you continuously notice positive changes in your behavior and thought patterns. Previously undreamed of reactions to food will become second nature. Armed with the effective tactics you'll learn from this book, you'll be prepared to face the enemy head-on, and like the title promises, conquer your cravings once and for all.

Introduction

Imagine a life where food cravings are a thing of the past. Imagine, if you can, a life in which:

- you can get through a whole evening at home without wondering if there's anything good to eat in the kitchen
- you can go to a party and be more interested in what the guests have to say than what's on the buffet table
- you're not afraid to take the first bite of your favorite food for fear you won't be able to stop eating until you've finished all of last week's leftovers
- you can be in the same room with a dozen doughnuts and not even be aware they're there
- you can take three bites of your Aunt Ruth's peanut-butter fudge and leave the rest sitting in front of you because you just don't want any more
- you can walk past a bakery window and not feel tortured to go inside and buy something
- you can say, "No thanks, I don't care for one" when your neighbor offers you one of her homemade chocolate chip cookies (and really mean it)
- you forget to eat

Do I hear laughter? If you're like a lot of people who obsess about food, you probably read this list and thought, "Yeah, right!" knowing those are things other people can do, not you. But admit it—in the back of your mind, didn't you secretly wish that list described you?

If that's the kind of relationship with food you've dreamed of but thought only other people had, you're waging your own private war with what you put in your mouth. Why are your cravings so bothersome? Because they lead you to do things you don't want to do or that you know will be bad for you. Your cravings compel you to eat when you're not hungry. They force you to consume snacks you don't need. They make you think you want a particular food, even though eating it would only make you feel worse. You feel that unless you give in to the urge, the craving won't go away, but when you do give in, the craving just comes back again. Your cravings make you feel like you're out of control around food, and they make you miserable.

Are you fighting this losing battle? You are:

- if you can't get through an hour without thinking about your next snack or meal
- if you live to eat instead of eat to live
- if you often eat unconsciously, unaware of how much or what you're putting in your mouth
- if you feel you can't resist food that's put in front of you
- if you rearrange the buffalo wings in the bucket so no one will notice how many you ate
- if you offer to clear the table just so you can eat the scraps in the kitchen
- if after one bite of a "forbidden food" you feel you've blown your diet and go on an all-out food frenzy
- if you feel you have no control over food and that food controls you

If you're sick and tired of the conflict, tired of being obsessed with eating, then it's time to stop struggling. You've been waging war with food and the cravings are winning, but don't surrender! There's nothing wrong with you. You're not sick. The only reason you're still struggling is because you haven't been using the right ammunition. How can you expect to win if you're not properly armed? How can you defeat the enemy if you're using the wrong tactics?

In this battle, if you think food is the enemy, you've been sabotaging yourself. Food is not the enemy—your erroneous thoughts are. These thoughts constantly bombard your brain and keep you trapped in the craving cycle, which goes like this:

- You have a negative thought.
- You experience anxiety and other unidentified negative emotions.
- You get the uncontrollable urge to eat.
- You experience added discomfort and anxiety as you struggle against the craving.
- You surrender and eat something.
- You feel bad for eating when you really didn't want to.
- You have negative thoughts about yourself.
- You feel even worse.
- You get the uncontrollable urge to eat.

And on and on it goes. No wonder the cravings never go away. This repetitious pattern will continue until you learn how to stop it and get off the treadmill.

Some steps in this cycle happen without you even being aware of them. You may not notice the thoughts that bring on your craving. In fact, you may not even notice the craving itself until you catch yourself with your hand on the refrigerator door.

From now on your number one priority is to attack your improper thought patterns and replace them with the kind of winning beliefs that will bring you the relief from your cravings that you long for.

Rather than fearing the next craving, you need to meet it head-on with an entirely new plan of action. If you're ever going to stop obsessing about food, you need to stop this destructive cycle dead in its tracks, preferably in its earliest stages. You need to recognize that the enemy is lurking right inside your head and call a halt to this nonproductive pattern.

This, you will soon learn, is the key to your strategy.

You may have discovered that cravings will sometimes go away on their own after fifteen or twenty minutes, but often twenty minutes is far too long to wait when fighting such powerful urges, especially if your habitual reaction to cravings is to give in to temptation and eat.

Rather than fighting a craving or trying to block it (an action that often intensifies the desire to eat), you can eliminate cravings altogether by following a simple four-step process. These steps are effective not only when used at the height of a craving, but also before one hits. The process is highly flexible, so you can tailor it to your particular needs. With practice, your cravings will occur less and less frequently, until you no longer fear them. Eventually, they will disappear almost completely.

The four steps work because they attack the very things that are keeping you trapped in the craving cycle:

- They cause you to become aware of the thought processes that have been leading to your cravings and show you how to turn them around in an instant.
- They help you identify the emotions your eating has been covering up.
- They introduce you to a powerful source of guidance that's inside you and is available to help you twenty-four hours a day.
- They teach you to treat yourself with kindness and respect, rather than undermining all your best efforts.

In these pages you'll read many things that are right on target. Over and over you'll find yourself thinking, "That's me!" There will also be some things that just don't click for you. That's okay. Try what feels right and stick with what works. There's something here for everyone who has ever fought a losing battle with food.

When thinking of your own inner struggle with the way you eat, you may be helped by this simple analogy: Picture for a moment one of those old war movies where a soldier is on guard duty near enemy lines. He's ever vigilant listening for the slightest noise. He paces back and forth with his rifle slung over his shoulder, ready for action. Suddenly, he becomes aware of an intruder.

What is the first thing he does?

He stands alert, and with a no-nonsense look on his face, takes aim in the direction of the noise, and shouts, "Halt! Who goes there?"

If you were the enemy lurking in the bushes, that would get your attention, wouldn't it? And that's exactly what you want to do. As soon as you become aware of your cravings, or the thoughts that led to them, you want to call a halt and focus your attention on the proper actions to stop your cravings in their tracks.

This is war and cravings are the enemy. When faced with a craving, you must learn to do what any well-trained guard does. When you fear the enemy is approaching, you stop it with that one simple word: HALT.

The four letters that make up this word represent the ammunition you need to conquer your cravings. Each letter signifies tactics that you can put to use on the spot to lessen your discomfort, banish your fears, and make your cravings disappear.

The HALT process is simple and easy to remember. As you'll learn in more detail, it consists of taking the following steps when you're facing the overwhelming urge to eat:

Hear your thoughts.

Allow yourself to feel.

Listen to your intuition.

Treat yourself lovingly.

These four steps offer a powerful method for stopping your cravings. They work best when followed sequentially, but you won't always need to use all four at once to get the desired result. There may even come a time when simply saying the word *HALT* to yourself will be enough to stop a craving!

Each step offers new ways of thinking, new ways of looking at yourself, and new ways of dealing with your problems, so when a craving hits, you'll be able to use whichever solution works for you at the moment.

As you learn to apply the four steps, you'll no longer struggle when faced with the overwhelming desire to eat. You'll learn cravings don't necessarily mean failure. With an understanding of the HALT process, you'll know exactly how to react. Instead of being something to fear, cravings will represent an opportunity to put your new strategy to work and succeed in ways you never thought possible.

Are you excited? You should be! You're in for a lot of new experiences. You're about to learn methods that will lead to major improvements in the way you relate to food. That does not, however, mean you'll no longer be able to enjoy your favorite treats. It doesn't mean you have to give up cake or pizza and start eating celery sticks for lunch. That's not the way the process works. Food is wonderful. Enjoying the incredible variety of delicious treats available is one of the great joys of living. You won't be asked to give that up.

Instead, you'll learn to deal with food in a healthy way and to eat without feeling guilty. The HALT process is about learning to enjoy all foods without obsessing about them.

And isn't it about time?

Part I
Hear Your Thoughts

1

Cravings and Thoughts

What is a craving? It's a gnawing, non-hungry need to eat that takes over your mind and blocks out all other thoughts. It's the feeling that the only thing that will make you feel better is food. It's an overwhelming, obsessive urge to consume, and the more you fight it, the stronger it becomes.

Sometimes the craving is specific, as in the desire for chocolate or something salty. It may be a craving for a particular texture, like creamy pudding or doughy pastry. Sometimes a craving is more general, giving the feeling that any food will satisfy it. But it's rarely satisfied for long.

Cravings can hit anytime and anywhere: when you're surrounded by friends or when you're alone, when you're tired or when you're energized, when you're overwhelmed with work or when you're bored, when you're calm or when your hormones are in an uproar.

Cravings are uncomfortable, bothersome, irritating, and often accompanied by the hopeless, defeated feeling of, "Oh no, here I go again."

It often seems as if the cravings control you.

If you give in to your cravings and eat when you don't really want to, you have to deal with the guilt and shame that often accompany overeating. This is usually followed by . . . what else? More cravings. It's a vicious cycle, but one that *can* be broken. It's really quite simple, and it all begins with your thoughts. Why? Because cravings are thoughts. Nothing more.

Because your cravings feel so powerful, it's easy to give them a life of their own. They can be so overwhelming, taking over all non-food-related thoughts, that it seems as if they're orders which must be obeyed.

The key to dealing with cravings is to realize that *you control your thoughts; your thoughts don't control you*. Because cravings are nothing more than thoughts, you also control your cravings, not the other way around.

People who have a problem with food often try a variety of methods to control their eating, including turning to diet pills. For someone who struggles with cravings, this will do no good whatsoever because most cravings hit when a person isn't hungry.

Suppressing your appetite with chemicals is not the solution.

Rather than controlling your appetite or what goes into your mouth, you need to control your thoughts. To do this, you need to first become aware of the difference between positive, empowering thoughts and the false or negative ones that bring on your cravings.

The first step in conquering your cravings (the *H* in HALT) is to *Hear* your thoughts.

You're bombarded with thousands of thoughts every day, either at a conscious or subconscious level. Your incredible computer-like brain is constantly processing sensory inputs and searching for the appropriate mental folder in which to place them. It files away everything you see— things you focus on deliberately and things you barely notice. It files away everything you hear—things that are said directly to you and sounds you pick up without even being aware of them.

Your brain can take the input from your nose and relate it to a strong childhood memory. This amazing organ does the same thing with taste, linking the signals it receives from things you put in your mouth to previously collected data about different foods. You may have thought an event or experience was long forgotten, but it had merely been filed away for safekeeping.

All this sensory input is compared with the stored information in your mental files to determine how you habitually react to a given situation. These thought files are what your brain uses to create your attitudes, beliefs, and most important, your actions.

Your craving thoughts are like a computer virus. Once they get in your brain's files, they spread to every folder, infecting all the data. To effectively fight your cravings, you need to access these files in your brain, especially the ones marked "food and cravings," and clean out that virus.

Until you become aware of what kind of data your brain is processing, you'll continue to behave subconsciously. You'll react out of habit, rather than taking steps to control your actions. By listening to what's going on in your mind, you can find out if your thought processes are working for or against you.

What are thoughts anyway? They're the voices of your many selves talking to you. This doesn't imply that you're schizophrenic or have multiple personalities. Your personality is made up of elements of all the roles you've ever played or experienced in your daily life. These roles each have their own voice, which communicates with you through your thoughts.

Inside you may be a parent, a child, a teacher, a judge, a lover, a guardian, and countless other characters. Depending on which of your selves is playing the leading role at the moment, the voice you hear in your thoughts may be loving and kind, or harsh and judgmental. The emotions this voice arouses in you will cause you to react a certain way. When you're struggling with a craving, you are subconsciously hearing some kind of negative voice.

It's absolutely essential, therefore, that the moment you become aware of a craving, you mentally call a HALT in your mind and take the first step to *hear* your thoughts. You need to bring your thoughts into your conscious awareness and find out what's really going on in your head. Find out what those voices are saying to you.

By calling a HALT, you instantly gain control of the situation. You've just stopped whatever thought initiated the craving, so you can now step back and hear what's going on inside.

Take this moment to ask yourself:
- What am I thinking?
- What triggered this craving?
- What do I need right now?
- What am I telling myself that's making me want to eat?

Knowing the answers to these questions puts you back in control. You're now behaving consciously rather than reacting to subconscious thoughts. Just like that guard on patrol, you can't fight the enemy if you're always sleeping on duty.

Stay alert, be vigilant, and hear your thoughts.

2
Triggers

Imagine this scenario: Mary, a young mother of two, is sitting in her favorite chair reading a book. She finished dinner less than half an hour ago and isn't the slightest bit hungry. Suddenly, out of the blue, a thought pops into her mind: "Go to the refrigerator." Accustomed as she is to responding to these kinds of thoughts, she obediently complies. She doesn't want to eat again so soon, but a craving has struck, and cravings must be satisfied (or so she's convinced herself).

Or how about another scenario: George, an insurance salesman, is sitting at his desk at work. He just finished a large lunch and ate more than he wanted. He's feeling somewhat uncomfortable, and more food is the last thing he needs, yet an all-too-familiar voice pipes up: "You need something sweet."

He doesn't stop to think about why he wants dessert. All he knows is that eating it will make the craving go away. Temporarily. George goes to the vending machine and gets a candy bar.

What happened? Neither of these people was doing anything that had to do with food. In each example, they'd recently eaten. Maybe they were even full, yet suddenly they had the desire to eat more. What brought on their cravings?

As you know by now, cravings are nothing more than thoughts. All thoughts are triggered by some kind of external stimulus. Becoming aware of your thoughts will help you find out what initially triggers your cravings. Once you're aware of your triggers, you can eliminate them, or if that's not possible, come up with a healthy way to deal with them.

Triggers can be verbal, visual, written, or some other type of stimuli. Food itself is a powerful craving stimulus and is probably the most obvious one. Who doesn't get the urge to indulge when smelling fresh-baked cinnamon buns or popcorn popping in the microwave?

Advertising executives are well aware of the power of triggers. Television commercials, magazine ads, and even billboards are deliberately designed to make you want to eat by prompting pleasant thoughts of eating. No matter how full you are, it's next to impossible to watch an ad for gooey, chocolaty Nestlé Toll House cookies without your mouth watering and your thoughts wandering to the kitchen cupboard. In fact, your mouth probably started watering just by reading about those cookies. This is physical proof of the power of written craving triggers.

Or, how about the visual image of a slice of steaming hot pizza being dished up, the cheese stretching from the pan to the plate? Even a mental image gets those gastric juices flowing, doesn't it?

These are the more obvious causes of your cravings, but have you ever stopped to wonder why you suddenly desire a snack when there's no noticeable trigger? You can be thinking about something that has nothing whatsoever to do with food, when suddenly a craving will hit.

The reason these less-subtle triggers can be so powerful is they affect you subconsciously. The thoughts you're aware of when you make an effort to hear them come from your conscious mind. Those that affect you more subtly (the ones that sneak up on you when you're not paying attention) come from those files buried way in the back in your subconscious mind. It's these unnoticed thoughts that are the most frequent cause of your cravings.

The subconscious part of your brain is a storehouse of everything you've ever heard or experienced. It remembers everything. Minor details you think you've forgotten are stored away in those computer-like files and will come drifting back to the surface, given the proper stimulus.

Let's take a look at Mary's and George's scenarios to see how this works. Mary was reading a book when her craving struck. If she had stopped to call a HALT at the instant she recognized the onset of the craving, she could have used that time to hear her thoughts and ask herself what triggered it. Not seeing or smelling any obvious food triggers, she might have thought to look at the last few sentences she'd read before the craving hit. If so, Mary would have been amazed to discover that the trigger was right there on the page.

Just before the desire to eat came on, she read the words, "Margaret looked in the mirror and hated what she saw." When Mary's brain read about a woman looking in the mirror, it found a match with a file on how Mary feels when she looks in the mirror.

What she read flipped a switch in her subconscious mind and brought on the craving. Without even being aware of it, Mary heard the critic voice in her head telling her that she didn't look so good. Because she wasn't aware that the words in the book had triggered her craving, Mary did the only thing she knew to quiet the subconscious thoughts in her head. She obediently put down the book and headed for the kitchen.

If she had taken the time to call a HALT at the moment she became aware of the voice telling her to eat, Mary would have realized there was no reason to obey her craving. She would have seen that she was not the character in her book and that she was not going to let some words on a piece of paper cause her to overeat.

Or how about the second scenario? George ate too much at lunch. His clothes were tighter at the waist, and he was finding it harder to breathe comfortably. On a conscious level he was barely aware of the discomfort, but subconsciously, a voice in his mind was telling him, "You ate too much. You're fat. Since you blew it again, you might as well eat some more."

George's brain translated these thoughts into a craving, and he responded by going in search of something to eat. If, however, he had taken time to call a HALT, he could have listened to the thoughts in his head. He would have realized that eating a little more than he intended for lunch wasn't the end of the world. By being aware of the cause of his cravings, he would have been in a position to take appropriate steps to deal with his discomfort, rather than eating even more. In this case, he might have responded by simply loosening his belt until the temporary fullness of lunch went away.

Awareness—hearing your thoughts and knowing what triggers them—is a key factor in understanding your cravings and heading them off in the future.

Exercise: Triggers

You can increase awareness of your cravings by generating a list of the things that may be causing them. You don't have to fill in all the blanks now. Wait until your next craving hits, then call a HALT and take a few steps backward to figure out what brought on the craving. Write your triggers in the following spaces as you discover what they are. It can be quite interesting and even amazing to discover some of the things that make you want to eat.

Visual triggers are things you see that make you want to eat. For example:
I saw a television commercial for ice cream.
I saw Jane in a bathing suit and remembered that mine doesn't fit anymore.

Write your own visual triggers here as you uncover them:

_____

_____

_____

_____

_____

Verbal triggers are remarks you overhear or things said to you directly. For example:
I heard John saying it looks like Sarah has gained a lot of weight lately.

Write your own verbal triggers here as you uncover them:

_____

_____

_____

_____

_____

Written triggers include phrases in books, signs, etc. For example:
I read a line in a novel that said, "The man handed him a candy bar."

Write your own written triggers here as you uncover them:

_____

_____

_____

_____

_____

Other triggers could include:
My clothes feel really tight.

Write your other craving triggers here as you uncover them:

_____

_____

_____

_____

_____

The next time you're hit with a craving, instead of instantly acting on it and grabbing something to eat, call a HALT. Do a little detective work and find out what triggered that craving. When you realize it was caused by a subconscious thought or an external trigger, you'll be able to create a deliberate and conscious reaction. Armed with this information, you may see there's no rational reason for you to act on your craving.

Always keep in mind that you don't have to eat a piece of cake just because a coworker brought it in. You don't have to eat the fresh bread just because it smells so good. These things may have triggered your craving, but cravings are only thoughts. In an instant, non-constructive thoughts can be stopped, turned around, and restated to your benefit.

3
Limiting Beliefs

Thoughts are extremely powerful. Unfortunately, most cravers have more experience with negative thinking than with positive, empowering thinking. How you deal with food is directly linked to the type of thoughts you choose to believe about food. In order to control your negative eating habits, it's vitally important that you recognize your limiting beliefs and understand how they affect the choices you make.

Every minute of the day your head is cluttered with thoughts. It's nearly impossible to block them our. Close your eyes for thirty seconds and try to erase all thoughts from your mind. Just relax and let your mind become a blank slate.

Could you do it? Chances are you were interrupted within a few seconds by your busy brain. Thousands of thoughts bounce around in there every hour, and these thoughts can have a tremendous effect on how you feel and how you act.

Despite the massive quantity of thoughts your brain is processing, most of them are actually quite consistent. People think the same kinds of thoughts day after day in an almost predictable sequence. Based on their mental files, they've programmed themselves to create specific thoughts in response to certain types of stimuli.

It's this kind of routine thinking pattern that you need to become aware of when dealing with food. By repeatedly hearing the same thoughts, you create your own set of deeply held truths, or beliefs, about yourself and the way you eat.

Your personal belief system is a result of a lifetime of programming—a lifetime of listening to what other people tell you, and more important, what you tell yourself. It's like being brainwashed. If a thought is repeated often enough, if you hear the same mental message over and over, you will begin to believe it, even if it isn't true.

Yes, that's right, even if it isn't true.

Once you start really listening to your thoughts, you may be surprised to discover how many of the beliefs about yourself that you regard as sacred truths are not only negative, but have no real basis in fact.

These false messages can be very damaging to your self-esteem. Rather than empowering you, they can cause you to think and behave in ways that are detrimental to your wellbeing—such as overeating.

If your subconscious thoughts are disapproving or critical, they can be sending you negative messages throughout the day without your being aware of their impact. Unless you're able to bring these messages to your conscious mind, they'll cause you a lot of unnecessary mental discomfort. For many people, this discomfort manifests itself as a desire to eat.

The good news is that even though you've allowed yourself to insert these negative beliefs into your mental files, it's equally possible to revise them, turning negative beliefs into positive, energizing ones.

So how do you start? Once again, by taking the first step and hearing your thoughts, becoming aware of the way you talk to yourself. Let's try another exercise to give you some practice.

Exercise: Limiting Beliefs

The following phrases are popularly held beliefs among people who suffer from recurring food cravings. If you have ever told yourself one of these phrases, make a check mark beside it. After you've gone through them, add your own beliefs that aren't on the list.

Beliefs About Yourself
_____ I have no willpower.
_____ I will never control my cravings.
_____ I am a failure.
_____ I can't stick to a diet.

24

Beliefs About Food

_____ I can't resist certain foods.

_____ I always overeat at parties.

_____ I can't get through the day without snacking.

_____ If I eat _____ (something fattening), I'm a bad person.

_____ If I blow my diet the whole day is a loss, so I might as well eat more.

Do any of these beliefs sound familiar? Which do you willingly accept as true about yourself? Chances are, if you believe they're true, you've never bothered to take the time to ask yourself *why* they're true. Many of them could easily be false, but you've programmed yourself to believe them, and you reinforce these beliefs every time they pop into your head and you don't refute them.

Go back over the list and look at each statement with a new and critical eye. Ask yourself why you believe it's true, then consider ways in which it might be false.

Let's look at a few examples:

1. If I blow my diet, the whole day is a loss.

Okay. Maybe you ate something that won't help you achieve or maintain your desired weight. Does that give you reason to continue eating and make matters worse? Why not look at this from a more positive point of view and consider what you didn't eat? Did you eat everything in sight? Did you then go to the corner deli and buy out the bakery section? (Even if you did, it could be worse.)

Chances are you ate a relatively small portion of a "forbidden" food before your craving for more started, brought on by your false "I've blown it" thoughts. If you had called a HALT and heard the way you were berating yourself for this minor digression, you would have reasoned that it could always be worse.

Punishing yourself by continuing to eat is not the answer. Once you realize that a minor setback doesn't mean the end of the world, you'll be able to use your awareness to stop yourself from making matters worse.

2. I can't resist certain foods.

Wait a minute. Let's look at this rationally. Can you resist eating liver and onions? Can you resist eating rotten eggs? If so, then there's no physical reason you can't resist *any* food, is there?

All food is created equal. It is nothing more than fuel: carbohydrates, protein, or fat that keeps your body running. So what is there to resist? If you look at a chocolate chip cookie as the lifeless blob of carbohydrates and fat that it is and realize that you are the one with the power, you'll see you've been subscribing to yet another false belief.

Yes, it's true. Certain foods like chocolate contain chemicals that make you temporarily feel better. The real reason you think you can't resist certain foods, however, is that you've given them power they don't possess. You've given away your power to an inanimate object. There is nothing to resist. Some foods may taste better than others. Some high carbohydrate foods may even give you a temporary physical high, but whether or not you choose to eat them is up to you. The food holds no magical power. It's all a matter of how you think about it.

How about one more?

3. I always overeat at parties.

Is this true? Always? Has there ever been a time when you went to a party and you ate just one plateful of food? If so, then your statement is false. Perhaps you usually eat more than you know is good for you at a party, but there's no physical reason you have to do so every time.

What if you were to tell yourself over and over, "I'm perfectly satisfied to eat just a little bit of a few things and stop"? Is there any reason this couldn't become your new belief? You chose to believe the original statement; why not reprogram your mind to believe something more healthy and empowering?

You can go back through all the false beliefs in the previous exercise and find a new and more positive way of restating each one. The same is true for every limiting belief you repeat to yourself countless times each day.

Changing the way you act is as simple as changing the things you tell yourself. Conquering your cravings can be as easy as changing your choice of words. Do your thoughts ever sound like this:

I can't resist chocolate.
I can't give up sweets.
I can't lose weight.
I can't control my cravings.

If these sound familiar, you not only tell yourself these things, you most likely believe them. You probably believe your thoughts so strongly that you've convinced yourself they are unchangeable character traits.

The problem isn't with your personality; it's with your vocabulary.

When you tell yourself you can't do something, your subconscious mind doesn't know if it's true or not. Your brain merely tells your body to act on the information you give it. Awareness of this fact is absolutely crucial to overcoming your cravings. If a voice inside you tells you over and over that you can't control your cravings, then you will act on that belief and let your cravings control *you*.

When you have a conversation with yourself, if you HALT for a moment and really listen to what you're saying, you can use that moment of reflection to consciously ask yourself:

Why can't I resist chocolate?
Why can't I give up sweets?
Why can't I lose weight?

You get the picture.

The answer is very simple: because you keep telling yourself you can't and you believe it.

Suppose you tell yourself, "I can't eat just one potato chip." If this is your belief, what will happen when you eat one potato chip? You will act on your belief and eat a second, third, and fourth potato chip. You may even finish the whole bag. Why? Because you've convinced yourself that for some reason other people can stop after one chip, but you can't. This is the type of limiting belief that will feed your cravings forever.

What if you were to suspend all disbelief for a moment and believe that you are capable of anything? What if you were to tell yourself that you *can* eat just one chip and stop? If you truly believe this, then you will eat exactly one chip and not want any more.

Sound too good to be true? The truth is: You can do anything you want to do. All you have to do is believe it. Believe this: if one other person on this earth has ever done the thing that you want to do, you can, too.

The solution to turning a negative thought into a positive one is as easy as hearing your thoughts in the first place, then changing their wording.

Changing the way you habitually talk to yourself will change your belief system, and the results will be immediate.

As you saw in the examples, one of the major ways you limit yourself is by using that nasty word *can't*. Remember the potato chip example? The only reason you couldn't eat just one was because you told yourself you couldn't and you believed it.

The reason you can't do something is not because you don't have the physical or mental ability to do it, but because you choose not to by the words you use. You can do anything you want, but by repeatedly telling yourself you can't, you make the subconscious choice to not even try.

Right now you may be telling yourself, "That's nor true. I've tried everything possible to lose weight (or to stop overeating, or to control my cravings), but nothing works."

The fact is, nothing will work until you change the way you talk to yourself. You may have taken every action you could think of, but you won't see results until you hear your thoughts and reword them to work for you, not against you.

When you tell yourself you can eat just one potato chip, that thought becomes your belief. You act on that belief, and you eat only one. You made the right choice based on your thoughts, and all it took was changing *I can't* to *I can*.

Exercise: Can Versus *Can't*

Think of the *I can't* phrases you habitually tell yourself about food, eating, or dieting. Be as honest as you can. As they come to mind, write them down, no matter how ridiculous they sound. (If you need more space, use a separate sheet of paper.)

I can't _____

I can't _____

I can't _____

I can't _____

I can't _____

Now go back over each sentence you wrote and cross out the words *I can't with* a big X. Next, rewrite the list, substituting *I can* for *I can't*. This may sound tedious, but the simple act of writing these new phrases will start the process of imprinting these new beliefs in your subconscious mind.

I can _____

I can _____

I can _____

I can _____

I can _____

Think about what you just wrote. is there any physical reason you can't do any of the things on that list? Of course not. Maybe the only excuse that really fits is that you've just never tried thinking that way before. Now all you have to do is believe what you've written. If any doubts pop into your mind, refuse to let them in. You *can* do it!

Reread your new sentences. You can actually feel the mood change they bring about, can't you? Notice how your thoughts affect your mood. Do you feel the positive lift that instantly accompanies positive thoughts?

How do the phrases you wrote affect the way you feel about yourself? As you learned when you read about the craving cycle, thoughts cause emotions. You should be able to sense the mood change your thoughts cause. Feel the hope and excitement that come over you just by changing that one word.

When you believe you can, your actions will follow. Starting today, make the choice to listen to the voices that talk to you in your thoughts. Hear the words you choose, and if they aren't working for you, change them.

From now on, any time you find yourself about to say you can't do something, HALT in midsentence. Hear your thoughts and acknowledge that when you really choose to, you can do anything.

You are not a victim. You may have been acting like one because of your erroneous thoughts, but every action you have ever taken is a result of a choice you have made. Every bite of food you put in your mouth is the result of a choice.

Who or what are you blaming for your cravings and reactions to them? Rather than remaining a victim of your choices, hold yourself accountable. Hear the thoughts that are leading you to make choices that may be detrimental to your well-being. Then take responsibility for yourself and turn your thoughts around.

If you feel yourself craving a food you know you shouldn't eat and you're really not hungry, realize that if you choose to do without it, you *can*. The choice is yours.

4
Affirmations

You've now seen how limiting beliefs and poorly worded thoughts work against you. Because you haven't stopped to hear your thoughts until now, you've unknowingly been causing your own cravings. Don't despair. You've also learned how by merely changing a few words you can turn a negative statement into one that empowers you.

The kind of positive statement you wrote in the second part of the *"Can Versus Can't"* exercise is an example of a self-help tool called an *affirmation*. Affirmations are upbeat sentences that lift your spirits and fill you with energy. They are the devices you can use to reprogram your erroneous belief system.

To change the data in your mental files, you'll need to come up with a list of affirmations to counteract your negative self-talk. By repeating this list over and over, either aloud or silently, you'll produce rapid changes in your habitual thought patterns. It's a highly effective way to clean out that craving virus from your mental files.

Affirmations are nothing more than positive statements about yourself or your situation. You've already seen how easy it is to write one type of affirmation by simply changing *can't* to *can*. In general, there are a few simple rules that should be followed if all your affirmations are to have the desired effect:

1. Write them down.

You're going to be repeating these phrases many, many times, and it's important to state them the same way each time. Also, the simple act of writing your new beliefs starts cementing them in your mind from the moment your pencil hits the paper.

2. Focus on yourself.

The majority of your affirmations should include the pronoun "I" plus a verb. This is all about making beneficial changes in *you,* so keep your focus right there.

3. Keep it positive.

This seems more than obvious, but you may discover a tendency to throw negative words such as *not, don't,* and *never* into your affirmations. This is a no-no. Using words such as *not* tends to make you focus on exactly what you don't want.

Take the following phrase as an example: "I am not fat." What image comes to mind? A fat person. To keep your affirmations positive, leave out those negative words. Write your affirmation like this instead: "I am thin."

This may seem like a ridiculous statement to make if you truly feel you're not thin. The important thing is that your affirmation will bring to mind the image of a thin you, which leads to the next rule . . .

4. Affirmations don't have to be true.

But you must want them to be. You believe what your thoughts tell you. When you believe something, you act on it and it eventually becomes true. 'This is how the entire set of negative beliefs you now hold has become your truth. By stating your desired outcome as if it were already fact, your actions will follow.

If you repeatedly tell yourself "I am thin," at some point when you reach for a doughnut, your brain will say, "Wait a minute. I am thin. Thin people don't eat doughnuts. Maybe something else would taste better instead."

See? Your brain acts on what you tell it.

If you don't believe this, just put an extra copy of your affirmations in a drawer for safekeeping. Some day in the future you'll be doing some spring cleaning and you'll come across them. If you've done your homework and really worked at reprogramming your beliefs, you'll discover the phrases you once thought couldn't possibly describe you, fit you to a tee.

5. Affirmations should energize you.

Choose words that not only make you feel good, but words that make you feel great. They should motivate you to run right out and do whatever is necessary to become a reflection of the person you are in your mind. If "I am thin" really empowers you, then use it. If "I have a terrific body!" revs you up even more, then choose those words for your affirmation.

By now you should have the hang of it, but let's use the examples from your list of food-related beliefs to come up with some good affirmations. Here's how the negative thoughts from that exercise can be restated as motivational phrases:

- *I have no willpower* becomes *I am strong and full of personal power.*
- *I will never control my cravings* becomes *I am learning strategies for dealing with cravings and am successfully using them to change my life.*
- *I am a failure* becomes *I succeed at things because I know I can.*
- *I can't stick to a diet* becomes *Diets are gone from my life because I now deal with food in a healthy manner.*
- *I can't resist certain foods* becomes *Food is just energy; I am the one with power. I choose what I will and will not eat.*
- *I always overeat at parties* becomes *I'm perfectly satisfied to eat just a little bit of a few things at a party.*
- *I can't stick to a diet* becomes *I choose to do without snacks if they make me feel bad.*
- *If I eat _____ I'm a bad person,* becomes *I am a good and lovable person no matter what I do or what I eat.*
- *If I blow my diet the whole day is a loss, so I might as well eat more* becomes *If I eat something that is not healthy, I make a conscious choice to eat better for the rest of the day.*

And there you have it. Simple, huh? They're written down and they start with *I* plus a verb. They are positive and full of motivating energy. They may not necessarily be true yet, but they reflect where you soon expect to be.

Each of these new affirmations should empower you. They should strike a chord and make you feel good about yourself. That's what affirmations are all about.

Use these affirmations as a guide to come up with your own list (Appendix B contains additional affirmations that may inspire you), and make a commitment to start reprogramming your belief system today. The first time you notice one of these new thoughts coming to mind instead of one of your old, false statements, you'll know you're making great progress.

But don't stop too soon. Remember, it took a lifetime of programming to imprint those tired old lies on your brain. It's been said that it takes three weeks of doing something new to break an old habit. Be prepared to devote at least that much time to making these phrases part of your new belief system.

This may seem like a lot of work, but using affirmations is not only painless, it actually makes you feel better as you do it. If your affirmations are worded correctly, you can't help but notice an improvement in your mood when you say them to yourself. If you've successfully rooted out the lies and misconceptions in your old, distorted thinking, you should have a list of new phrases that make you feel terrific.

You'll need to do whatever it takes to make your affirmations part of your new life. There are a variety of ways to make this easier:

- Keep a list by your bed and read it first thing in the morning and last thing at night before you turn out the light.
- Tape a list to your bathroom mirror and repeat your affirmations as you brush your teeth.
- Write your affirmations on three-by-five-inch cards and read them anytime you have a free moment, such as while waiting in line at the bank or grocery store.
- Print them on Post-it notes and stick them on your desk, on your steering wheel—anywhere you'll be sure to see them.
- Make a tape recording of yourself reading your affirmations. Listen to it while resting in your favorite chair or before going to sleep.

These phrases should become so familiar to you that any time a craving hits, you can HALT your negative thinking and replace it with your new positive thoughts. Now that you're starting to use your new strategies, you can add a couple more affirmations to your list:

- I discard my old, worn-out beliefs as I hear them.
- I am building the life I've always dreamed of.
- I am conquering my cravings with my powerful thoughts!

5

Self-Esteem

One of the least recognized craving triggers is also one of the most common: low self-esteem. When the mind quietly whispers, "You are worthless," or "You are unlovable," the craver doesn't want to hear it. She responds by stuffing down those frightening voices with food. In this situation, food serves as both a source of temporary comfort and as a punishment for her perceived deficiencies.

Think back a few pages to the story of Mary. Her desire to run to the refrigerator wasn't caused by a real need to eat. Her craving wasn't brought on by the smell of food or the sight of dessert. Instead, a sentence on a page triggered Mary's low self-esteem, even though she wasn't consciously aware of it.

When she read the sentence "Margaret looked in the mirror and hated what she saw," Mary subconsciously thought about how she also hated what she saw every morning when she looked in her own mirror. Rather than face her dissatisfaction with herself, Mary's self-protective mechanism kicked in and directed her to find something to eat.

Low self-esteem in cravers can be the result of many factors, but a poor body image is one which most people who struggle with food share. If you were to listen to what you habitually tell yourself about your size and shape, would you find that you are helping or hurting your self-esteem? Is what you're telling yourself about your body only making you want to eat more?

There are a lot of Marys out there who can't stand looking in the mirror. The reflection that looks back at them doesn't match up with their desired image. It taunts them and tells them, "You're not good enough."

This kind of self-defeating, self-deprecating attitude is understandable in today's society. Americans are obsessed with body size and beauty. We are barraged daily with images of "the perfect body" from countless sources. Television ads portray the average housewife as slim and trim. Magazine covers show beautiful, pencil-thin women in skin-tight dresses next to titles that shout, "Take It Off and Keep It Off!" or "Have the Body a Man Would Die For." Is it any wonder the diet industry is raking in billion of dollars a year?

Television shows with female stars flaunting picture-perfect bodies in hide-nothing bathing suits do nothing to improve the morale of the majority of American women who wouldn't dare be seen in a bikini. We're never told about the horrific diets these models have to follow to maintain their sleek profiles. We never hear that many of them suffer from eating disorders.

Instead, media and television only reinforce the idea that thin is in. Those who buy into this concept falsely believe skinny people enjoy life more. They think thin people have more fun, more friends, more energy, and better clothes. They believe they have the best partners, more self-confidence, and more money.

In other words, if you're not thin, you miss the boat. Ironically, this false belief leads many people to drown their dissatisfaction in milk shakes.

Low self-esteem is often inversely related to body size. In other words, the higher one's weight, the lower one's self-esteem. People who are insecure about their body size fight a constant struggle to lose or maintain their weight in order to live up to an image of the ideal body. They spend a lot of time thinking about food, yet they feel out of control around it. They obsess about how they eat and how they look.

If an honest and objective appraisal of your body shows you really are carrying around some extra pounds, you should realize your excess weight may be the external result of internal turmoil. You are hurting on the inside, and this is being reflected on the outside with an extra layer of insulation.

If you fall into this category, you really can't blame yourself for being dissatisfied. You are a result of society's programming. If, however, your dissatisfaction has led you to become preoccupied with what and how you eat to a point that makes you unhappy, some changes are in order.

Are thoughts about the way you look only adding to your cravings? If so, the place to begin is with a self-image make-over. Think about it: people go to department stores or spas for makeovers to improve their external appearance when they should actually pay more attention to what's going on inside.

An image makeover begins with your thoughts. Therefore, begin with this one: You are the same lovable, worthy person whether you weigh 120 pounds or 320 pounds. Your number one goal should be to become a self-satisfied person, free of cravings and accepting of yourself, *no matter what you weigh.*

Your makeover can address every aspect of your self-image, not just how you look, but since poor body image is a common denominator of most cravers, we'll start there. The last couple of chapters rooted out some of the limiting beliefs you hold about your behavior around food. Now think about some of the beliefs you have about the way you look. How might these be causing your cravings? Do any of the following sound painfully familiar?

I am fat.
I am ugly.
My thighs are too big.
My nose is too flat.
My hips are too wide.
My stomach is too soft.
I have no chest.

What a depressing list! Eating a jelly doughnut would definitely be more pleasurable than facing thoughts like those. But it sure wouldn't help things in the long run. By applying the principles of positive self-talk, which you have already tried and are having success with, you can make mental changes that will ultimately result in physical changes as well.

Unfortunately, certain physical characteristics are fixed and permanent. For example, changing your thoughts isn't going to change the shape of your nose. Changing your thoughts can, however, improve the way you feel about yourself in general, and that's a step in the right direction.

Take a few minutes to complete the following questionnaire, which is designed to improve your awareness of how you see yourself.

Exercise: Body Image

Complete the following statements.
1. When I look in the mirror, I feel:_____
2. The part(s) of my body I am most dissatisfied with is (are): _____
3. I am dissatisfied with my body because: _____
4. If I could change something about my body, I would change: _____
5. I would make this change because: _____
6. The part(s) of my body I am most satisfied with is (are): _____
7. I like this (these) part(s) of my body because: _____

Was this exercise difficult for you? Why? What reactions did it cause? Most important, what are you telling yourself as a result of answering the questions?

HALT!

By any chance, do you feel the urge to eat now? Why? Hear your thoughts and notice if doing this exercise raised any voices that may have triggered a craving. If so, this area could use some mental housekeeping.

If a poor body image is causing you to feel less than beautiful on the inside, the key to improving your self-concept is through the process of self-acceptance. Accepting your body is the first crucial step in raising your self-esteem. It comes before changing the way you eat. It comes before starting an exercise program. Self-acceptance is the first step in loving yourself.

Nathaniel Branden is a well-known expert on self-esteem. In his book *How to Raise Your Self-Esteem,* he explains that by accepting yourself you do not have to be happy with the way you look. You are only asked to accept the way you are at this very moment. You simply need to learn to look in a mirror and say, "Okay, this is the way I am right now."

Think about the way you see your body. Do you immediately focus on certain parts that you dislike? Maybe you take the opposite tack and refuse to even think about the parts you're unhappy with. Instead of accepting yourself, you may actually be rejecting parts of yourself.

So you don't like what you see in the mirror? Accept that what you see is the way you are, rather than denying your shortcomings. Then accept that you have the power to change those things about your body or appearance that you feel need changing.

There may be some things you would like to change, and with the proper determination and motivation, you have the power to do so. There will also always be parts of you that can't be changed. The way to be at peace with all of your parts is to accept yourself as you are.

You may resist the very thought of self-acceptance. You may be thinking, "Oh, no. I can't stand myself right now. I am unacceptable."

As long as you continue to reject yourself as you are, you will not be receptive to change. You will be stuck in a rut, fighting your thoughts, and triggering endless cravings. The more you deny something, the more it will cause you problems.

As Branden stresses, by accepting yourself, you are not admitting that you don't have any imperfections. In doing so, you are simply ending your struggle with yourself. You are opening yourself to the possibility of change. You are giving yourself a starting point from which to move forward.

Take control of your life. Hear your thoughts. Throw out the ones that drag down your self-esteem, and take responsibility for yourself. You are not a victim of the voices in your head.

To get a better feel for how well you accept yourself, think about how you react when people compliment you on your looks. If you deny or refuse their compliments, hear your thoughts and ask yourself why you have trouble accepting what they tell you. If you don't believe people are telling you the truth when they praise you, there are parts of yourself you are denying. Unless they have ulterior motives, people who give compliments are usually being sincere. Listen to your thoughts and find out why you have a hard time believing or accepting the good things other people see in you.

It's also useful to examine how accurate and current your view of yourself is. When you picture yourself, or even when facing yourself in the mirror, do you see yourself as you were years ago, rather than how you actually are today? Were you a gangly teenager with a bad haircut? Was your weight different then than it is now? If you've changed physically, has your mental image changed with you? If not, how is this helping or hurting you? Try to see yourself without blinders or ghosts from the past.

Besides having a poor body image, there are other indicators that can signal low self-esteem: You may not feel worthy unless you have others' approval. You may have a nagging feeling of being inadequate, as if you can never live up to others' expectations. You may not feel you're good enough, without even knowing what "good enough" is.

Your self-image, like your belief system, comes from things other people have been telling you all your life, as well as things you've been telling yourself. If you grew up in a loving, supportive home, your sense of self-worth will be much higher than someone who was raised in a household filled with negativity and put-downs. Women, much more than men, don't value their own self- worth as much as they should. They are caretakers, spending more time worrying about how other people feel than about how they feel. They give more love to others than to themselves.

Unfortunately, if you don't love yourself, you won't feel as loved by others as you really are. It's hard to accept love when you don't accept yourself or feel worthy of love. In the absence of love, it's too easy to turn to food to fill the void.

That void can be filled by accepting yourself as you are. Again, this doesn't mean you have to like everything about yourself. You simply accept that you will work with what you've been given. Doing this allows you to identify what you'd like to change and move forward from there.

Ask yourself what things you do that cause you to like yourself less. What routine behaviors do you disapprove of? Accept that this behavior is a result of your belief system. Then take a good, hard look at yourself and determine what you'd like to change. Understand your motivations for wanting to change. Is it to please someone else or to please yourself? As you begin to do things for yourself, as you take charge and make positive changes rather than remaining a victim, you will see a corresponding increase in your self-esteem and a decrease in your cravings.

In what ways does your behavior around food make you unhappy? Can you accept that this behavior is a result of poor mental programming? Now that you understand that, are you willing to make the effort to change your behavior? The more you take responsibility for yourself, taking charge of your actions and your life, the more you will begin to like yourself and stop turning to food for comfort.

Exercise: Labels

The following sentences will help you identify the words you use to describe yourself. Check those that fit your image of you as you see yourself today, then add your own in the blank spaces provided. Remember, learning to love yourself can be a painful process, but it has tremendous rewards. You can begin now by accepting the way you are at this moment, whether you're happy with yourself or not.

____ I am dumb.
____ I am lazy.
____ I am sloppy.
____ I am friendly.
____ I am caring.
____ I drink too much.
____ I am athletic.
____ I eat too much.
____ I am tone-deaf.
____ I am good with kids.
____ I am bad with numbers.
____ I can't cook.
____ I can't sing.
____ I am too needy.
____ I have a food problem.
____ I am too impatient.

Now add your own:

_____

_____

_____

The phrases you checked and those you wrote in add up to form your self-image. They are examples of the labels you use to identify yourself.

Were there any you didn't particularly care for? If so, why have you continued to hang on to them?

If your goal is to conquer your cravings, one of the most important labels to eliminate is the one that says you are a person who has a problem with food. You can get rid of this identity by simply accepting the situation. Stop fighting it or denying it. Then, if you're sick and tired of the way you deal with food and don't want to struggle with cravings for the rest of your life, decide to make a commitment to do everything within your power to change whatever behaviors are causing your cravings. If you no longer want to consider yourself someone with a food problem, find a new label for yourself that you like and take whatever action is necessary to make it describe you.

You can eliminate your cravings even faster and improve your self-esteem tremendously by changing all the other labels you're not happy with. Get rid of descriptors that don't help your self-image by creating a new vision of who you are. Perhaps you've always wanted to learn to play the piano, but your parents couldn't afford lessons when you were younger. What's keeping you from pulling out the yellow pages right now and finding a music teacher? Or maybe you always wanted to be able to draw, but the people you sketch look like figures in a game of hangman. Why not take an art class at your local community college?

Creating a new image for yourself, complete with new labels, can change your entire concept of who you are and what you're capable of. The sky's the limit! First, accept that the list you created in the "Labels" exercise represents who you are right now. If you're not happy with anything on it, what's keeping you from taking responsibility for your life *this very moment* and creating The New You?

Every January 1, millions of people make New Year's resolutions. They identify something they don't like about themselves and come up with a plan to make it better. Why wait until the new year? Why not make your own list of New You resolutions? Get fired up about something other than food!

- Finish your degree.
- Learn a new language.
- Write the book that's in your head.
- Learn to play the clarinet.

- Become computer literate.
- Design your own home page on the World Wide Web.
- Take a psychology class.
- Start an exercise program.
- Run a marathon
- Become a volunteer.

By creating a new focus in your life, you will redefine yourself. You will no longer think of yourself as a person with a food problem. As your focus changes, your thoughts will change with it.

Making lifelong, permanent changes in the way you see yourself takes a dedicated effort. You'll need to reinforce yourself every step of the way. One way to do this is by starting each day with a "motivational moment." Take a minute before you get going in the morning and focus on the things you like about yourself. Praise your positive attributes. Give thanks for the things about yourself that you're proud of. Make up a little "I love me because" speech and incorporate your most empowering affirmations. Most important, take this opportunity to emphasize that you are a worthy, lovable person.

Do this 365 days a year and you will be healing yourself with a giant dose of self-love. After all, your happiness isn't determined by how much you weigh or how your clothes fit. It's not measured by how much or how little you eat. Your happiness is determined by how you feel inside.

Continue to listen to your thoughts as you take responsibility for your actions. Every change you make on your own behalf will cause your self-esteem to climb. The higher your self-image, the better you can handle anything life throws at you and the less you will turn to food for comfort.

Part II
Allow Yourself to Feel

6

Feelings

The initial step in the HALT process works because it attacks that crucial first stage of the craving cycle: negative thoughts. By themselves, negative thoughts aren't so bad, but unfortunately, if you listen to them, they inevitably lead to the second stage in the cycle: negative emotions.

At the first sign of anxiety, most cravers immediately think of food. They don't like dealing with the cause of their cravings, so they eat instead. If overeating and struggling with cravings is no longer an acceptable option for you, if you don't want to put up with the torment anymore, you're going to have to deal with the things you've been avoiding. The second step in the HALT process, therefore, is to *allow* yourself to feel.

You may find this concept somewhat strange. Of course, you know how you feel during a craving. You're anxious and uncomfortable. That's why you want to eat so badly—to make the anxiety go away and to feel better.

Before you can truly feel better, however, you need to understand that the anxiety you experience during a craving isn't the cause of the craving. This is actually a secondary emotion that has forced its way into your consciousness. The discomfort you experience during a craving is the result of any number of underlying needs and emotions that, just like your thoughts, you may not even be aware of.

Often these more basic feelings are too painful to deal with. Primary emotions such as fear, anger, and guilt can be so unpleasant that most people would prefer not to face them at all. That's why the phrase, "Don't worry—be happy" caught on so quickly. It capitalized on the nearly universal desire to feel good rather than deal with the normal ups and downs of life.

Human nature being the way it is, the easy alternative to experiencing negative emotions is to find ways to suppress them or make them go away. Unfortunately, far too many people have become experts at doing just that. Alcohol and tranquilizers provide an escape from painful feelings for some, but for others doughnuts and pizza offer the same refuge from life's problems. To a compulsive overeater, food is a drug. The pleasure of biting into a sugary candy bar or a doughy pastry can temporarily blot out mental distress better than any painkiller.

If cravings are a recurring problem for you, it's likely you've been using food to protect yourself from pain. Do you use food as a drug, eating to insulate yourself from your feelings and needs? It may be hard to admit, but food can be abused just as easily as alcohol. The problem is, you have to eat to survive.

With all of the social rituals surrounding what we eat, it's easy to ignore the fact that food's main purpose is to fuel our bodies. We grow up equating food with pleasant times such as special meals with family, birthday celebrations, and parties. Think about the times your mother gave you a cookie to make you feel better when you were upset, or the warm feeling of sitting at the Thanksgiving table, filling your stomach with turkey, stuffing, and pumpkin pie while surrounded by people you love. Events like this psychologically link food with comfort and feeling good.

Yes, food is fuel, but it has undeniably evolved into more than that. It's an integral part of our culture. What would a wedding be without cake? What would a baseball game be without hot dogs? Food plays a central role in most social events and holidays. It's even present at many business meetings.

If food were consumed only to sustain life, there would be no demand for junk foods that have no nutritional value. The rows of chips, cookies, and other snack foods in grocery stores show us that food has become much more than just a source of energy. If you consistently use food to feel good, to comfort you when you're feeling down, or to relieve boredom, stress, loneliness, or fear, then you are eating for other than social reasons or to provide your body life-sustaining energy.

If you've been putting food in your mouth as a way of stuffing down your feelings, you may not realize how you have numbed your emotions so much that you only allow yourself to feel good. Better advice than "Just say no" to food is to HALT and allow yourself to feel. Rather than blocking your emotions artificially with food or any other substance, experience those you've been trying so hard to suppress.

Cravings are a protective mechanism. They shield you from experiencing negative feelings. If you respond to cravings by eating, you never have to face the underlying emotions that caused the cravings in the first place. Rather than turning to food when you get a craving, you should acknowledge this anxiety as a sign that your thought process is out of whack and making you feel bad. Your craving should signal that there's something you're not allowing yourself to feel.

Think about it. If you always felt good, you would never experience cravings. Picture those times when you experience strong feelings of happiness, fulfillment, or joy. You may still enjoy the good taste of a favorite food, but when everything is going well, you just don't experience the same overwhelming, relentless urge to eat.

If you've ever experienced the heady exhilaration of a new relationship, think back to how good you felt. All was right with the world, wasn't it? If you had been paying attention to your body and your thoughts, you most likely would have discovered that your cravings had diminished or even disappeared.

The excitement of a new romance brings on such a range of good emotions that people who have struggled with cravings for years can suddenly find themselves craving-free for months. This is because the intoxicating initial stages of a romantic relationship block out negative emotions. Your basic human needs are being met and the majority of your emotions are positive. You are so filled with love that there is no need to use food as a substitute for feeling good.

Unfortunately, when the initial high of new love fades, it leaves room for the normal range of positive and negative emotions to surface, and cravings reappear. Unless you have learned how to successfully deal with these feelings, you'll fall right back into the habit of using food to mask your anxiety.

If your habitual reaction to uncomfortable feelings is to medicate yourself with food, any negative emotion can bring on a craving. It doesn't matter what the feeling is about since cravings occur to protect you from discomfort of any kind.

It may seem strange that to eliminate your cravings you have to make a deliberate effort to experience exactly what your cravings are trying to protect you from. Unfortunately, if you continue to suppress your feelings by giving in and eating every time a craving hits, you'll never get below the surface and be able to deal with the real problem.

By following the second step in the HALT process and *allowing* yourself to feel your negative feelings, you will help eliminate your cravings. If you allow yourself to experience all of your feelings, negative as well as positive, you'll be able to discover what's at the root of your cravings and find ways to deal with them more productively.

Rather than immediately turning to food for comfort, you will try to resolve your problems by facing them instead of blocking them from your consciousness. Once you learn to turn to yourself or others to help you feel better, you'll no longer experience the overwhelming urge to turn to food as the solution to your problems.

While it may sound hard to suggest that you suddenly start feeling what you've been trying to avoid for years, keep in mind that it's not possible, nor desirable, to feel good all the time. Your negative emotions serve a purpose. They compel you to change. You can learn valuable lessons from your difficulties. It's often the most challenging times in your life that give you the opportunity to grow.

By not allowing yourself to experience your pain, you never give yourself a chance to be complete. If you make the effort to HALT during a craving, to hear your thoughts and allow yourself to feel the emotions that make you want to eat, you will discover parts of yourself you have been hiding or denying.

You must feel things you've become an expert at not feeling. The process may be difficult. It requires conscious effort. It isn't easy to break old habits and go through the steps. But if you're sick and tired of fighting cravings, if you don't want to struggle with food one more minute, then you'll be willing to make the effort to do the mental work necessary to conquer your cravings.

7
Needs

Everyone eats in response to physical hunger. There's no denying when you're really hungry. Your stomach feels empty. It growls and rumbles, telling you to feed it. You may even feel shaky or irritable. This is the body's way of telling you it needs nourishment.

Cravers, however, eat in response to a different kind of hunger. This hunger isn't from a lack of food. It's a nonphysical desire for something that food will never feed. It's emotional hunger—the need to fill some human desire that isn't being met.

People with low self-esteem experience more cravings than those with high self-esteem because one of their most basic needs is not being met: the need for love. They don't love and accept themselves as they should and they feel unworthy of accepting love from others. To fill this void, they turn to food.

All humans share the same basic emotional needs. In addition to the need to be loved, we need to be nurtured, to be accepted, and to experience joy and peace. There are other needs that can be added to this list in varying degrees, depending on the individual, such as the need for understanding, for attention, for independence.

Cravers often ridicule themselves for a lack of willpower around food when, in fact, their overeating is more a result of not dealing with their normal human needs and desires. Any excess weight most likely stems from unresolved inner issues surrounding love, nurturing, and other unmet needs rather than from a lack of self-control.

In order to know if your hunger is physical or mental, you must allow yourself to feel. When you become aware that you're craving something to eat, call a HALT and ask yourself, "Why do I want to feed myself now?"

Before you move to the more subtle internal issues, start with the basics. Review your physical needs. Allow yourself to feel your body by asking yourself:

- Am I really hungry now?
- When was the last time I ate?
- What did I eat and how much?
- Should I be hungry again already?

This last question is especially important because not all foods are created equal when it comes to how long they'll satisfy you physically. Was your last meal a small snack or an all-you-can-eat buffet? Equally important as how much you last ate is *what* you ate.

Fruits and vegetables stick with you only about one hour. That's why you get hungry so quickly after eating Chinese food (it's mostly veggies). Starches such as bread and pasta last a little longer, up to two hours. Proteins such as yogurt or chicken are the longest lasting, providing energy for as long as four hours. Think about what you last ate and ask yourself if your hunger is valid.

If you routinely give in to your cravings, you probably don't ever go more than a few hours without eating something. Experiencing real physical hunger may be a rare occurrence for you. If so, it's very important that you HALT and allow yourself to feel your body's hunger instead of eating in response to nonphysical needs.

If you evaluate what and when you last ate and allow yourself to feel your body's hunger signals, you may find you're not hungry at all. Perhaps you're just exhausted and have mistaken tiredness for hunger. If you have the desire to eat, but tuning in to your body shows you're only mildly hungry, then it's time to find out the real cause of your appetite.

The whole issue of real hunger versus psychological hunger is why diet pills are not the answer for people with cravings. Chemicals only attack the physiological side of overeating. They take away the feeling of true hunger. They do nothing to deal with the underlying emotional issues that plague cravers.

Sure, you may lose weight temporarily while using diet pills. Chalk that up to willpower and the effect of trying something new. But what happens when you go off the pills? You're left with the same unresolved issues. The pills haven't done a thing to address the problems your cravings mask and before long you return to the same eating patterns as before.

Using food as a substitute for love, nurturing, attention, or any other need does not work. These things come only from within, not from some external source. Food is not love. Food is not comfort. it may have been used as a replacement for these things when you were a child, but as an adult it's up to you to fill these needs in other ways. The way you were raised and the way you learned to deal with food as a child can give you some valuable insights into why you deal with food as you do now. Take a few minutes to complete the following questionnaire, it's designed to increase your self-awareness, a necessary tool in your fight against cravings.

Exercise: Food Assessment

Think about the following questions and write out your answers in detail. The insight you gain will help identify what may be holding back your recovery from food obsession.

1. What are your fondest memories while you were growing up?
2. What are the most difficult memories from your childhood?
3. Did food play a part in any of these memories?
4. At what age did you become aware of your preoccupation with food?
5. How did you become aware it was a problem?
6. What was going on in your life at that time?
7. How did you feel about yourself then?
8. Was your eating a response to those issues?
9. Are the same issues that brought on your preoccupation still affecting you today?
10. How did eating make you feel at that time?
11. Does food still have the same effect on you now? Explain.
12. What kinds of rules surrounded food as you were growing up? (For example, did you have to clean your plate at every meal? Were you allowed to snack between meals?)

13. Do you still apply those rules to yourself?
14. Was food used as a reward? If so, for what?
15. When are you most likely to get cravings now?

This exercise should show you how the majority of your eating habits and attitudes were formed when you were young. Even though you may have changed in many other ways, your childhood eating habits may still control your actions today. They may also be standing between you and the kind of relationship with food and your body that you want and need. If this is the case, this increased awareness can help you make more informed choices, allowing you to break old habits and rules that no longer serve you.

You can start by identifying your strongest needs. Go back to the previous exercise. What situations that have nothing to do with food usually bring on your cravings? What is lacking in your life at those times? Are you feeling ignored? Deprived? Unloved? Allow yourself to feel your needs. It's only by identifying the real cause of your cravings that you'll be able to heal yourself and stop obsessing about your next snack. By continuing to eat when you're not hungry, you are leaving legitimate needs unrecognized. As long as they remain submerged, they will bump around inside you, causing all kinds of damage. The fallout from your frustrated yearnings is an assortment of negative emotions.

Instead of allowing these negative emotions to manifest themselves as cravings, accept your needs as legitimate and commit yourself to taking appropriate action to feed your soul, not your stomach.

8

Guilt, Shame, and Other Bugaboos

Sarah is an office manager for a large department store. Her husband, Jim, is a salesman who is on the road a lot. They have two children. In spite of the fact that Jim likes the way she looks, Sarah isn't happy with her weight. She's always trying one diet or another and describes herself as a "closet craver." Food is a major issue in Sarah's life, but her family has no idea how much it occupies her thoughts or how unhappy she is because of her cravings.

What follows is a typical day in Sarah's life.

It's Wednesday and Sarah is disgusted with herself. She's done it again. She told herself she wasn't going to overeat. She ate too much after dinner for the last three days and went to bed every night feeling nauseated. She woke up this morning with a food hangover. She felt groggy, bloated, and depressed, just like she did when she went to bed. She didn't care if she never ate again.

Sarah was determined to do better this time and felt she started out pretty well. She ate a small but healthy breakfast. She didn't really want to eat, but everybody always said breakfast was the most important meal of the day.

At work she was especially good. She walked by the candy machine four times and only hesitated for a moment. There was no way she was going to touch that stuff. Not today. Not ever again. No more bingeing.

Lunch was a salad with fat-free dressing at the deli near the store. She gave a fleeting thought to buying those big cookies by the register for dessert, but today was her day to quit, so she was strong. She opened her desk drawer for a mid-afternoon snack, but was afraid if she opened that new bag of pretzels she'd finish off the whole thing. She shut the drawer and gave herself a mental pat on the back.

She was good at dinner, too. Everybody else went back for seconds, but Sarah was a real trooper. No bread. No butter. She didn't even clean her plate. She left a couple of bites, just like all the magazines said she should.

Then she blew it. Big time. Jim and the kids went their separate ways and left Sarah to clean up. There she was clearing the table. Without even thinking, she nibbled a bite of meat loaf Jim had left on his plate. No one was around, so she had more. She felt a slight twinge of something in the back of her mind, but hey, that meat loaf tasted even better than it did at the table.

Little alarms started going off in her head, but she blocked them out and cleaned up the rest of the plates. Literally. Never mind the fact that she'd been so good all day. Never mind the fact that she'd left food on her own plate just a few minutes earlier. This was different. She was only doing the dishes, and besides, calories don't count if you eat standing up, right?

The kitchen was as clean as it was going to get. There wasn't a dirty pot or pan in sight. The others were off doing their own things, so like every other night, Sarah settled in on the couch to watch television. Okay, she may have eaten some stuff back there in the kitchen that she didn't mean to, but she told herself not to think about it. She didn't want to deal with that now. She pushed all thoughts to the back of her mind and stared at the mindless sitcom on the screen.

Time for a commercial. No, she didn't want to take a break. She wished they'd put the show back on so she wouldn't have to think about anything. She'd made cookies for the kids on Sunday. Weren't there some left in the jar?

"No, you're not going to do this to yourself again," she thought.

Good, the show was back on. It didn't seem very funny tonight. Okay, just two cookies. She knew she could stop at two, and besides, they were fat free. She went to the kitchen, took only two cookies as she'd promised herself, and returned to the couch. There, see? She'd done it. Just two cookies.

"They sure didn't last long," Sarah thought. Did she even finish that second one? She couldn't remember. Maybe she had set it down. She looked around, but it was gone. The cookies had disappeared much too quickly. She told herself two more wouldn't hurt. She knew she could stop at four, but Sarah worried that if she had two more, somebody might notice how many were missing. Maybe if she rearranged them in the jar nobody would know the difference.

She went to the kitchen a second time, as if on automatic pilot. As she reached for the cupboard where the cookies were, she glanced at the trash can and saw a pizza box from the kids' lunch. She knew they always left the crust. No, she thought, she wouldn't stoop that low ...

Sarah is under food's spell. After a full day of denying her feelings and fighting with herself, she is giving in to the powerful lure of her cravings. Her control is slipping away faster than she can reel it in. She resisted the desire to overeat all day, but now she's losing her grip.

What is Sarah feeling at this point? She has more negative emotions boiling inside her than she's even aware of. If she were to single out the feelings she's experiencing, the list would probably surprise her. It would include self-loathing, depression, disappointment, fear, shame, and guilt. Lots of guilt.

Where do these feelings come from?

The self-loathing comes from telling herself she's a failure. Sarah promised herself she wasn't going to overeat again, yet she caved in and repeated the same pattern she falls into night after night. She is disgusted with herself for being so weak. She knows how she wanted to deal with food but believes she showed no self-control whatsoever. She's depressed because she feels she's fighting a losing battle. She has convinced herself she's overweight and unattractive. She's let herself down again. She's disappointed that she didn't have the willpower to go through just one evening without bingeing.

She's afraid she's going to be miserable forever, battling with food for the rest of her life. She's terrified she's going to get fat. She's worried about losing control. She's afraid other people are going to find out what she's really like.

She's ashamed of stooping so low as to eat leftover food off other people's plates. She's embarrassed at how she uses doing the dishes as an excuse to eat in private. She's appalled at the thought that she would pick food out of the trash can.

All of these things make her feel guilty. She has so much guilt she might as well have a neon sign over her head flashing, "Guilty! Weak person! Guilty! Failure!" She may not have identified what she's feeling as guilt. All she knows is she doesn't like it. She wants it to stop so badly she's turning to the one thing that will only make it worse: more food.

It's easy to see where Sarah's guilt comes from. She has devised her own set of rules about food and eating. Everything she does and everything she eats is either "good" or "bad." If she sticks to her rules, she is good. If she doesn't, she isn't just bad, she is a bad *person*. Her self-imposed list of shoulds and shouldn'ts becomes the focus of all her actions, as well as the criteria by which she judges herself.

This laundry list of negative emotions is directly related to Sarah's cravings. She's doing an excellent job of blocking them when they first appear, then stuffing them down with food.

If Sarah were to HALT and allow herself to feel, what other emotions might be underneath the food-related ones? What needs might Sarah have that she's not allowing herself to experience?

Sarah is bored with her job and with her life. She's tired of the same old routine of working every day and doing nothing but watching television in the evenings. She knows she's smart, but she never finished her degree once the kids came along. She's frustrated that she's not doing as much with her life as she knows she's capable of. She may have the vague sense that she's not fulfilled, but she stuffs that feeling down so quickly with food that she's not fully aware of the problem. Unfortunately, as long as she continues to respond this way, she will never take time to figure out how she could become more fulfilled, nor will she take the action required to follow through on what she learns.

Sarah doesn't know it, but she's also angry. Jim isn't home that often, but when he is, he spends all his time in his workshop. And where are the kids? Why couldn't they have helped her clean up? Why does everyone disappear right after dinner and leave her all alone? Maybe part of it is her fault, but she won't let herself think that far.

As if all this weren't enough, Sarah is also feeling lonely and rejected. Her basic needs for love, attention, and companionship aren't being met.

Jim may have his own reasons for needing privacy, but if the two of them are having problems, they aren't going to be addressed while Sarah sits on the couch night after night watching TV and snacking.

Perhaps as you read over Sarah's problems, some easy solutions come to mind. Sarah, however, can't see them. She has become an expert at numbing her emotions. They are buried so deep below the meat loaf and cookies she can't even begin to deal with them.

Some of Sarah's needs and feelings are perfectly valid. Others aren't completely reasonable. Unfortunately, all of them will continue to affect her until she allows herself to feel them, hears what she's telling herself, and takes action on what she learns. In the meantime, she'll continue to act on her negative thoughts. She'll continue to use the television as a distraction and food as a tranquilizer so she doesn't have to deal with the turmoil in her life and in her head.

Sarah's story may be painful for you to read. If you've struggled with food cravings, some of her actions may hit a little close to home. Hopefully, reading about Sarah has opened your eyes to the causes of some of your own eating problems. Guilt was one of the major feelings Sarah wasn't facing. Are you like Sarah in that you label yourself and all your actions either good or bad? If so, you are setting yourself up to fail. With the first bite of food that you don't really need, your guilt alarms will go off. Everything else you do after that may be a direct result of your guilty feelings. Recognizing the cause of your actions is the first step in erasing your guilt about overeating. Everything you do has a purpose. You may act and react in ways that are detrimental to your health and well-being, but it is always with the goal of protecting yourself from pain or discomfort.

When you eat something you think you shouldn't have, it's okay to be angry or disappointed with yourself, but you should take the time to ask yourself why you ate in the first place. Hear your thoughts and allow yourself to feel what led you to put that food in your mouth. Eating was a conscious choice on your part, even if the cause was subconscious. What feeling were you trying to feed? What need wasn't being met?

Once you allow yourself to feel what was going on inside your head before you binged, you will see that your eating was a self- protective mechanism. That doesn't make it right. That doesn't mean you can't be angry with yourself for turning to food for relief. But it does show you can take another course of action next time.

Instead of letting guilt eat away at you, release your guilt by accepting your actions and taking responsibility for them. Channel any anger or disappointment you may feel into a positive force. Use it to spur you on to action. Anger can be a very strong motivator.

Once you hear your thoughts and identify your feelings, you can determine what in your life needs to be changed. This may be an easy fix for a short-term problem, or it may call for a long-term solution for more complicated issues. It may require you to make some major life changes. All you have to do is ask yourself if you're satisfied with your life.

Ask yourself if you're happy with the way you're handling your problems. If not, then use any guilt you've had in the past to your benefit. Think of your old eating habits as a sign that something needed changing. Your guilt and your cravings have served their purpose, but you don't need them anymore. It's time to take responsibility and take action.

In dealing with the needs and emotions that have caused your cravings, realize that your negative feelings are valid emotions that need to be heard. It's impossible to be happy all the time. Accept your unhappiness, dissatisfaction, and any other negative feelings as normal and expected. Instead of suppressing them as you have in the past, admit that it's normal to have them. Once you've accepted them, however, relax and simply let them go.

Letting go of your negative thoughts and emotions can be as easy as imagining them flowing through you like driftwood floating on a river. Instead of damming the negative thoughts in that river, visualize them peacefully flowing right through you. Instead of being afraid of them and reacting to them with tension, recognize and release them!

What kinds of fears are you holding onto that are helping to maintain your cravings? Fear can be a good thing. The fight or flight syndrome that fills you with adrenaline when you face a dangerous situation can save your life. The fears related to food and eating, however, are often unwarranted and cause nothing but problems.

Rather than leading you to find safety, craving-causing fears will only lead you to behave in ways that are detrimental to your well-being. If you don't allow yourself to feel your fears, the anxiety you experience will continue to churn inside you, perpetuating your cravings. You will look for safety and comfort in eating. Food will act as your security blanket. The solution is to root out your fears and face them head-on.

There are any number of fears cravers try to mask: fear of failure, fear of looking foolish, fear of rejection, fear of criticism. Perhaps you're afraid of losing control. Perhaps you're afraid others will find out how much you really eat and won't think well of you. Maybe the thought of making changes in your eating habits or lifestyle is intimidating to you.

The best time to work on your fears is when you're not actually having a craving. By recognizing the false fears that routinely plague you, you'll be better prepared to combat them when they actually trigger a craving. As with other emotions, most of your fears are a result of erroneous thinking. Identifying what is making you anxious can, in most cases, be all that's necessary to reduce your apprehension.

Many fears are caused by rampant "what ifs." You may want to make positive changes in your behavior, but constant worry about the outcome may be standing in your way. Your what ifs may include:

- What if I get rid of all the snacks in the house and then I get hungry?
- What if I want to eat a small bowl of ice cream after dinner and end up eating a whole pint?
- What if somebody at the party comments on how much I'm eating?

In many cases you can ease your anxiety with positive self-talk. Take time to think through all potential outcomes if the situation were really to occur. Cover all possibilities, no matter how outrageous they seem. You may well discover that your fears are unfounded, or at least aren't as bad as you imagine them to be. The situation might not arise in the first place, but if it did, it probably wouldn't be the catastrophe you imagine.

There will be times when your fears are valid. If this is the case, and something truly bad could happen, knowing in advance what outcomes you may face will prepare you to deal with the situation with foresight. Forewarned is forearmed. You'll be facing your fears instead of dangerously covering them up with food.

Whether or not your fears are valid, rather than suppressing them, accept that they exist. Just like other feelings you've been stuffing down with food, until you accept them, you will fear your fears. Until you allow yourself to feel them, they will continue to control you.

Your fear or unwillingness to experience your feelings is what keeps your cravings coming back. Happily, once you begin to fully experience your fears, they will go away. By allowing yourself to feel all your emotions, and then accepting them, you will no longer fear them. You will be in control of your mind and your actions, not the other way around.

Let's use Sarah's story as an example of how you can use acceptance to deal with your emotions.

Sarah had two categories of emotions to deal with. In the first category were all of the negative feelings that were directly related to her cravings and the overeating that resulted from giving in to them: self-loathing, depression, fear, shame, and guilt. To clear out these feelings, Sarah could tell herself:

- I accept that I'm not happy with myself tonight because of the way I ate. I have every reason to want to kick myself. Now I can either sit here and continue to eat, or I can figure out what else is bothering me and do something about it! Or:

- I accept that my eating is out of control. I accept that I did some things I consider shameful related to my eating. I behaved that way in response to other things that are going on in my life. I'm really tired of feeling and acting this way. I am going to make some changes so I don't react this way anymore.

Next, Sarah can deal with the second category of negative feelings— those that were the original cause of her cravings: (Adapted from the guilt-clearing exercises in *How to Raise Your Self Esteem* by Nathaniel Branden, Bantam Books: New York, 1987).

- I accept that I'm bored and frustrated. It's no wonder I feel this way when my job is so routine and all I do is watch TV every night. I accept responsibility for the fact that I allowed myself to get to this point. I know I have the intelligence and ability to do much more with my life. I will come up with a plan to be more fulfilled so I don't feel the need to turn to food. Or:

- I accept that I'm angry with my family and with myself, and that's okay. Now I can either sit here and continue to let my anger and loneliness contribute to my weight, or I can do something about it!

Just like Sarah, you, too, can take responsibility for your feelings and for your actions. Hear your thoughts, then allow yourself to feel what emotions your thoughts are causing. Ask yourself what feelings you tend to suppress with food. What would happen if you brought these to the surface?

It can be very hard to face your feelings. You may find yourself wanting to shout, "I don't want to feel this way. I hate being this miserable!" or "I don't want to be lonely. I'd rather eat than feel like this."

Remember: even that kind of reaction is valid. Accept the way you're feeling, then ask yourself if you want to struggle with cravings for the rest of your life. Ask yourself if you want to stay trapped in the craving cycle, covering up those miserable feelings with food, all the while feeling even more miserable with yourself for the way you eat. If the answer is an emphatic "No!" take responsibility for your life and take action to deal with whatever is causing your cravings.

9

Conscious Mental Dialoguing

Facing the negative emotions you've been stuffing down may seem like a daunting task, but don't forget about the power of your own thoughts. By using your imagination, you can make your thoughts work for you through a process called *conscious mental dialoguing.* This simple yet effective technique will increase your self-awareness and help you identify and deal with negative emotions.

Remember how your thoughts manifest themselves as various voices, such as the child, the critic, the parent, or the teacher? In a conscious mental dialogue you deliberately create another voice that is extremely helpful in allowing yourself to feel: the counselor.

Of course, the counselor is really just another side of you, but until now you may not have taken advantage of this helpful part of your personality. Like a real therapist, the counselor is the side of you that takes time to listen and helps you analyze what's going on inside. Unlike the subconscious voice of a craving, it's the counselor's job to guide you in process of facing and feeling your emotions consciously, as they occur.

Before learning how to dialogue with your counselor voice, let's first examine how you talk to yourself during a craving when it remains strictly at the subconscious level. Picture your inner struggle as a cartoon where there's a little devil with a pitchfork sitting on your shoulder whispering nasty messages in your ear.

The devil represents the voice of your craving (pretty accurate analogy, isn't it?). He's urging you to do things you really don't want to do and is trying to sabotage all your good efforts.

In the following example you'll read a dialogue that is probably pretty close to the subconscious mental dialogue that goes on in your mind during a craving. Notice the struggle. It's like a tug-of-war between the craver and the voice of that little devil:

DEVIL: Hey! You ate too much for lunch. Why stop there? Why don't you eat something else? A candy bar would taste real good right now.
MARY: Oh no. Not again. I just ate .
DEVIL: Boy, did you ever! And your clothes feel really tight.
Go ahead . . . eat some more!
MARY: But I don't want to!
DEVIL: Of course you do. A candy bar will make you feel great.
MARY: No, it won't, and it'll make me fat.
DEVIL: What's the difference? You're already fat. One more candy bar isn't going to hurt.
MARY: But I won't be able to stop after just one.
DEVIL: Sure you will. Go for it.
MARY: No! I won't give in this time. I'm not going to go to that vending machine.
DEVIL: Oh yes, you are. You're weak. You can't resist that junk food. Why don't you just admit defeat and eat the candy bar. It'll taste so good.

And on and on it goes. Did you notice how many limiting beliefs and poorly worded thoughts were in that one, short mental conversation? This craver is not listening to her thoughts at all, nor is she allowing herself to feel. What emotions was she aware of? Mostly anxiety and despair, but little else. She made no effort to get beneath the surface of her thoughts and find out what was causing them. All she did was struggle with the voice of the craving. You can guess who won this confrontation.

Unfortunately, by remaining at this level of inner dialoguing, this craver didn't change a thing. The battle in her head will continue relentlessly until she gives in to the craving and eats the candy bar. Even worse, the next time she trips one of her craving triggers, she'll have the same kind of conversation all over again. It truly is a vicious cycle.

In a *conscious* mental dialogue, you direct your counselor voice to dig into your subconscious mind by asking probing questions and listening to the facts. You analyze the situation objectively. There's none of the judging and blaming that accompany a typical conversation with your craving voice. Based on objective questioning, you make unbiased observations and suggestions, which is something you probably haven't been doing too much of if you've been stuffing down your emotions with food. Remember, if you suffer from recurring food cravings and respond to them by overeating, you're out of touch with your emotions. In order to allow yourself to feel them, you need to make a deliberate effort to become aware of what they are and what's causing them. Calling on your counselor voice and deliberately carrying on a conscious mental dialogue will help you do this.

The moment you recognize a craving, instead of letting subconscious thoughts determine your actions, you first bring them to the surface by hearing them. Then you can allow yourself to feel the emotions they cause by having a mental conversation as if you were your own counselor.

You don't need to be a trained psychotherapist to do this. It's actually quite easy and you can have fun with it. Picture a patient lying on a couch with a counselor seated beside her in a big, leather armchair. What does the counselor do? She asks a lot of questions and takes notes. You've probably seen plenty of funny shows where the therapist talks something like this: "So, tell me what happened to make you upset? I see, and how did that make you feel? Ah yes, and how do you feel about this now? Mm hmm. . . and how does it feel to feel like that?"

If you could read the patient's mind, she's probably thinking, "And they get paid for this?"

In all seriousness, this kind of repetitive, systematic questioning serves a purpose. It requires the patient to look deep inside and find her own answers. And that is exactly the purpose of a conscious mental dialogue. By deliberately using your counselor voice, you greatly increase your awareness of your thoughts and feelings and come up with your own way of dealing with them. In a dialogue with your counselor, you simply direct your thoughts for a specific purpose—in this case, to work your way past a craving to the negative emotion that caused it.

If this all sounds a little ridiculous, answer this: has what you've been doing so far worked to stop your cravings? If not, then why not keep an open mind and give it a try. When you dialogue with yourself, pretend you're your own counselor. Ask yourself probing questions to discover what the craver inside you is feeling. Allow your counselor side to systematically examine your feelings. You need all the information you can get to analyze the situation and come up with a better way to deal with your feelings than eating.

Don't let your counselor make any judgments. You should remain as objective and rational as possible. Dig at your emotions, asking as many questions as it takes to get below the surface to their root cause. Take a step back and see things you haven't allowed yourself to see.

Now let's look at a second craving situation and see what happens when you call in your counselor. We'll start out the conversation again the way most cravings start—at the subconscious level:

DEVIL: Hey! You ate too much for lunch. Why stop there? Why don't you eat something else? A candy bar would taste real good right now.
MARY: Oh no. Not again. I just ate. Won't these cravings ever stop?

In the back of her mind, the craver recognizes that she's struggling. This is where a light bulb goes off over her head and she remembers to call a HALT. Now that she's stopped the craving in its tracks, she decides to be her own counselor and carry on a conscious mental dialogue.

COUNSELOR: What's going on? What were you just thinking?
MARY: I don't know. I just got this overwhelming urge to eat something.
COUNSELOR: Well, you don't have any reason to be hungry since you just ate lunch. So what thoughts were running through your head?
MARY: Well, I guess I was thinking that once again I ate too much for lunch.
COUNSELOR: I see. So you're feeling a little angry with yourself. Did you really overeat? You had soup and a bagel.
MARY: Yes, but now I'm full and my clothes are tight.
COUNSELOR: OK, so you agree that you really didn't eat too much. Your clothes are temporarily uncomfortable because your stomach is full. What are you telling yourself about that?
MARY: My clothes are too tight because I'm fat.

COUNSELOR: Your clothes will feel better in a little while, after you've digested your meal. Meanwhile, when you tell yourself you're fat and that you overate, how does that make you feel?

MARY: I feel like a failure. I just can't lose these last few pounds.

COUNSELOR: I see. So you're also feeling a little bad about yourself. What else are you feeling?

MARY: I'm afraid I'll start eating and not stop until I feel sick.

COUNSELOR: Hmm. So you also feel a little fear that you'll lose control.

MARY: Yeah. I guess so.

COUNSELOR: Other than the discomfort from your tight clothes, how does your body feel right now?

MARY: Well, I feel tense and my stomach is in knots.

COUNSELOR: OK, that's because you're struggling against the craving. Let's look at this situation objectively. Do you agree that you really did eat a good lunch?

MARY: Yes.

COUNSELOR: What could you have eaten for lunch that really would not have been good for you?

MARY: Any number of things. They had a plate of cookies in the dining room, but I passed them up.

COUNSELOR: Aha! So you certainly didn't overeat. in fact, you did something you don't normally do. Is there any reason you can't pass up a snack right now?

MARY: Well, I don't know. I always give in .

COUNSELOR: Listen to what you're telling yourself. You don't always give in. It's only when you stop believing in your own power and tell yourself you can't do something that you give in. You can easily say no to a snack. There's nothing to be afraid of.

And there you have it. This conversation can be continued for as long as it takes to ease the craving. Did you notice how the counselor stayed completely objective? She didn't judge the craver and tell her how silly she was for feeling the way she did. She simply listened, then probed for the emotions beneath the surface. She identified a little anger, some insecurity, fear, depression, and even a touch of shame. She then pointed out the incorrect thinking and turned the situation around, showing more positive ways of looking at things.

Look at how the craver made the shift from a subconscious dialogue to a conscious and deliberate mental dialogue with her counselor voice. All it took was an awareness of the fact that she was having a craving. She immediately called a HALT, allowing herself to follow the first two steps of hearing her thoughts and becoming an objective observer of her situation.

See how easy this is?

When you talk to yourself in the middle of a craving, you choose which voices are in control. There's no reason for the craving voice to remain in charge when you direct your thoughts. Shift to a position of power by knocking that little devil right off your shoulder and conversing with your counselor.

Here's another example, and once again, the initial conversation during a craving takes place at the subconscious level:

DEVIL: Hey! Look at the secretary's desk! She brought in a dozen doughnuts! Why don't you go take one or two of them?
MARY: Oh no! I'm doing so well on my diet.
DEVIL: Aw, forget that self-righteous diet nonsense. Those doughnuts are just what you need to get through the morning.
MARY: I hate this. Now I'm going to sit here and crave those doughnuts all morning.

(Alarm bells sound in her head.) HALT! She realizes it's time to call in the counselor and shift to the conscious dialoguing mode.

COUNSELOR: What's going on? What were you just thinking?
MARY: Hmm. I was thinking that somebody is always bringing junk food into the office and I'll never be able to eat the right things.
COUNSELOR: OK, how did that make you feel?
MARY: I guess I felt kind of hopeless. Yeah. Defeated.
COUNSELOR: Why is that?
MARY: Well, I guess I feel weak around that kind of food. I just can't resist it.

COUNSELOR: Watch out for that word "can't", Mary. What else were you feeling?

MARY: I don't know. Maybe I thought eating the doughnuts would make it easier to get through the morning.

COUNSELOR: Oh, I see. So maybe you were feeling a little bored, too?

MARY: Yeah, come to think of it, I guess I was.

COUNSELOR: Well, let's take another look at this situation. People bring food into the office all the time. Do you always eat it?

MARY: No, sometimes I'm too wrapped up in what I'm doing.

COUNSELOR: There! You don't always eat the goodies. Those are just doughnuts. They don't have any power over you. You have the power of choice. You did it before and you can do it this time. Is eating the doughnuts going to make the time go any faster?

MARY: No.

COUNSELOR: Okay. So you are not weak and powerless. On the contrary. You are powerful. Look at that box of doughnuts and smile because they hold no power over you. How do you feel now?

MARY: Much better!

COUNSELOR: Why?

MARY: Because I took back my power. I'm in charge again. Now maybe I can get some work done.

What a contrast! Before Mary became consciously aware of the craving, she was only minutes from heading straight for those doughnuts. Once she recognized what was happening, however, she called a HALT and consciously called in the counselor.

Notice how, once again, the counselor remained totally objective. Unlike the craving voice that was quick to berate the craver and goad her into going against her better judgment, the counselor made no accusations. She asked questions designed to make her think and feel. She didn't stop with just one emotion, but probed deeper to uncover any underlying issues.

With the help and guidance of her counselor, Mary discovered that underneath the surface anxiety were several other thoughts and emotions she hadn't been aware of: helplessness, low self-esteem, and even boredom. Because she allowed herself to feel these emotions, she was able to deal with them quite easily by simply turning her thoughts around. As in the first example, the outcome was highly positive: not only did the craver not give in to the craving, but the desire to eat disappeared and was replaced with a renewed sense of power and hope.

Just by reading these two examples you can feel the difference in results between a subconscious conversation and one in which the victim of a craving really pays attention to what's going on in her mind. In the subconscious dialogues, the craver was only aware of the surface-level anxiety, rather than the underlying thoughts that usually accompany cravings. She knew she really didn't want to eat, but instead she struggled with her craving voice over the same old issue: should I eat or shouldn't I?

If she hadn't chosen to call in her counselor and carry on a conscious mental dialogue, she would have responded to the craving in her habitual way. In the second example, the conversation started out the same, but look what happened when she recognized the craving and remembered what to do. Despite being afraid of failure, despite a little bit of panic over having a craving, she remembered to call a HALT. She took back her power.

To stop a craving, you need to make a deliberate and conscious effort to call on your own counselor. When you halt your normal craver's dialogue, you'll be able to regroup and try another strategy rather than remain a victim.

10

Visualization

Now that you've seen how dialoguing works, you can plan ahead and be prepared to do the same type of therapy on yourself the next time a craving hits. The actual dialogue is quite easy. Often the hardest part is recognizing when it's time to call on your counselor and initiate the mental conversation.

One way to prepare yourself is through a process called *visualization*. You may already practice visualization in other aspects of your life. If you've ever performed before an audience or played in a sport, chances are you visualized your performance ahead of time, running through every scene or movement in your mind. That was visualization. This kind of mental rehearsal gives you confidence when it's time to actually play the role or perform the task because you've already done it, if only in your mind.

Visualization is extremely helpful in dealing with cravings. By anticipating and practicing the conscious reactions you've learned for combating your cravings, you'll be prepared to deal with them instead of falling back on your habitual patterns of response. As with any new skill or knowledge, the strategies in this book need to be practiced and applied repeatedly until they become a natural response to a given situation. The following exercise will show you how to imagine a scenario in your mind and give you a chance to practice some of your dialoguing skills, using the visualization technique.

Exercise: Visualization

Read the entire exercise and familiarize yourself with the procedure before attempting the visualization.

Choose one of your craving triggers from the list you came up with in the chapter on triggers. Now that you know the particular issue you'll be working on, choose a place where you'll be uninterrupted for a short while. Eliminate any distractions by turning off the television or radio (you can play some soft music if you find that relaxing). Sit or lie in a comfortable position and close your eyes. Take several minutes to breathe deeply and consciously relax every part of your body, one part at a time, moving slowly from the top of your head to the tip of your toes.

Try to let all of the busy thoughts in your mind flow through you. If an unwanted thought occurs to you, simply let go of it and continue to calm your mind and body. When you feel completely relaxed, complete the following steps very slowly in your mind:

- Picture yourself in the trigger situation you've chosen. You are in the grip of a very strong craving. All you want to do is eat.
- Visualize your surroundings . . . Where are you? What are you doing? Are you alone? What has happened to trigger your craving?
- Imagine how your body feels. Are you tense? If so, where do you feel the tightness?
- Identify the thoughts running through your mind. How do those thoughts make you feel? Afraid? Panicky? Hopeless? Recognize that this is the voice of your cravings.
- Now imagine yourself realizing that you are struggling with a craving, but you are in control. Become aware that this is an opportunity to use your new strategies.
- Hear yourself calling out "HALT" in your mind. Mentally put out your hand, signaling a stop to your craving. Feel the power that comes from taking charge. Feel excitement replace fear as you recognize the chance to succeed and conquer this craving.
- Begin to encourage yourself. What do you say?
- Picture yourself brushing aside the craving voice and refusing to listen to its negative messages.

- Now that you're fully aware of your thoughts, call on your counselor to talk you through the craving. Imagine the conversation you will have with her. Think of the feelings she may uncover.
- Practice talking to your counselor until she has uncovered all of the layers of emotions underlying your craving. Hear her words of encouragement. Know that you believe what she says. Work together to experience the emotions you've been blocking.
- Feel yourself responding to the inner dialogue with a renewed sense of power and hope. Feel your fears disappearing along with your craving.
- Imagine yourself moving on to an activity that is enjoyable, with no thoughts of food or failure.
- Enjoy the relaxation that flows over you as the tension disappears. How does your body feel? How do you feel about yourself? Enjoy these feelings and images until you are ready to open your eyes. You should feel refreshed and energetic.

Simply reading through the exercise is not enough to prepare you to use your new strategies. For the best results, you need to actually rehearse the steps in your mind. If you've never before done this type of exercise, set aside any reservations you may have and try it. What do you have to lose? At the very least you'll be relaxed and rested when it's over. You'll probably even finish with a smile on your face.

An added bonus of visualization is that the subconscious brain often can't tell the difference between an actual occurrence and an imagined one, so your visualization will become one more success in your battle against cravings. If you walk yourself through the steps, the thoughts and actions you imagined will become a positive reinforcement that your subconscious will store away to call upon in the future.

Because you've now practiced your reactions to a trigger situation, the next time you find yourself having the kind of craving you visualized, the very images and conversation you rehearsed in your mind will come back to help you through the real thing. That's putting your subconscious to work for you.

Training and preparation are critical to success in your battle, so practice visualization for any type of craving situation you're likely to encounter. Do this as often as you need to until you're confident in your ability to recognize when you're having a craving, call a HALT, and bring in the counselor. Know the types of questions your counselor needs to ask. Become familiar with objectively analyzing all your emotions. You want these things to become second nature.

The more confident you become in your ability to apply your new tactics in the face of an attack, the more your fear of cravings will diminish. That sinking feeling you experience now when you recognize a craving will change from "Oh, no!" to "Okay!" because you have a plan and you know how you're going to react.

Now that you're hearing your thoughts and allowing yourself to feel, steps three and four in the HALT process will show you additional ways of dealing with the feelings you've been ignoring for so long but are now learning to face. Since you'll no longer be turning to food as a way to make you feel better, you'll learn alternative methods that are far healthier and will bring you the peace of mind you deserve.

Negative feelings aren't nearly as intimidating when you begin to face them. Once you shine the light on your emotions, they can't hide in the shadows and cause you anxiety any longer.

Part III
Listen to Your Intuition

11

The Voice of Reason

By following the second step in the HALT process, you are bringing your feelings to the surface. Unfortunately, your between-meal snacking may still be hidden. Before you let that old guilt nag at you again, rest assured that you aren't alone.

Many cravers are sneak-eaters. Most of their snacking occurs when no one is looking. The shame of feeling so out of control pushes them to eat most snacks secretly so no one will notice how often or how much they eat.

Because of their embarrassment, most people who obsess about food not only eat in secrecy, they suffer in silence. The shame of feeling so out of control is hard to admit. Even those closest to a craver are often unaware of how troublesome their cravings are. It doesn't help matters that isolation and loneliness only exacerbate cravings.

You may think no one else understands the way you feel. Unfortunately, because others with the same problem don't want to confess to their own obsession with food, you may mistakenly believe you're the only one who's suffering. If you were to share your experiences, however, you'd find that your thoughts and behaviors are actually quite common. There's no shortage of people who have felt the same fears, the same shame, and the same sense of failure that you are working to overcome.

How many people know the extent of your preoccupation with food? Is your struggle with cravings something you talk about with family and friends, or do you try to handle your problem alone? Those who are still trying to eliminate their food obsession, as well as those who have already conquered their cravings, can be a tremendous source of encouragement and support in your struggle to succeed. Now is when you can use that kind of support more than ever. Changing old habits and dealing with unaccustomed emotions can be intimidating, especially if you think you have to deal with all this on your own.

There's no need to worry, however, if you're not ready to go public. You may be fighting the enemy, but you aren't the Lone Ranger. You actually have a reliable and confidential source of support that can be your greatest ally in combating cravings.

In fighting your personal battle, you are like a commander with your own aide-dc-camp. This source of help and guidance has been with you all along, but you may not have been aware of it. Like all military aides, yours is unfailingly loyal and dependable but stays out of your way until called upon.

You see, there's a part of you that instinctively knows what you need to do to get past your cravings. It's always aware of your feelings—probably much more so than you are at this point. This part of you can provide answers to questions that are otherwise beyond your ability.

If you doubt its existence, you just need a touch of imagination and a little trust. If you're the kind of person who doesn't believe anything until you can see it, feel it, touch it, or taste it, you may need to be a little flexible here. You'll never have physical proof that your personal aide exists. Once you experience the way it can help you with your cravings, however, you won't have any doubts.

In fact, you may have already been aware of its presence from time to time but didn't realize what you were dealing with. Think about it: Have you ever been sitting at an intersection, waiting for the light to turn green, and when it did a little voice inside you said, "Don't go yet"? You'd been all set to hit the accelerator, but instead of charging ahead, you hesitated. The pause was just long enough to see a truck barrel through the intersection, right where you would have been if you hadn't listened to that little voice.

Or perhaps you remember a time when something told you to go to the bedroom, even though you'd just come from there and everything was in order. You acted on this feeling and went back to find that the iron had fallen over and was burning a hole through the ironing board.

Chance occurrences happen often enough that we can all recall events for which we have no rational explanation. In these two examples, along with many other seeming coincidences, that voice is actually your own inner source of guidance, which you probably know as *intuition*.

The existence of intuition or an inner guiding force can't be proven. You can't see it, taste it, or touch it. It's more a feeling than anything concrete. Some people are much more tuned in to it than others, but this skill can be developed. In the meantime, you just have to trust that it's there.

Trusting your intuition is like being a passenger on an airplane. People who might be uncomfortable letting someone else drive them on the highway think nothing of putting their lives in a pilot's hands for a flight. They may be a little apprehensive about flying, but if they want to go somewhere badly enough, they'll get on board, putting their full faith in the pilot to safely get them where they're going.

If you've ever flown, you put your trust in the pilot. You trusted that he or she had the proper experience and the right qualifications. Because you had faith in his or her abilities, you were able to sit back and relax.

Learning to have faith in your intuition is like that. You may not be able to see it, but you only need to trust that it's there in order to begin benefitting from it. When you tune in to your intuition, you'll recognize what a tremendous source of support it can be in conquering your cravings.

Intuition is more than just a fleeting thought that tells you to take a particular action. It's a source of guidance from within that has access to more knowledge, facts, and insights than our rational, earthbound minds can tap into. Call it what you want. Call it your inner guide, your higher power, your soul, or your spirit. Call it Gertrude if you want. What you choose to name this guiding force is up to you, but recognize it as a friend who is there to help you.

Just like an aide you can call on at all hours, your intuition is also always at your disposal. Imagine the possibilities! While you may be restricted by your human physical and mental limitations, it's encouraging to think there's a part of you that isn't hindered by boundaries.

The experience of Terry, a college student from a small Midwestern town, illustrates the benefits of communicating with your intuition. Not only did Terry find out she had an inner guide who was listening when she needed help, but she learned that this all-knowing source had the answer to a question that had evaded her for years.

Terry had a nice figure and appeared to eat well, so her friends had no idea that she'd struggled with cravings for years. Because she appeared happy and content with herself, no one would have guessed she was so unhappy on the inside.

Terry felt like her eating was out of control. Every time she got a craving for food, she would panic, fearing her normal reaction of giving in to the craving and overeating. She felt that food controlled her life, but she didn't know what to do about it.

One evening, Terry had been studying in her dorm room when she was overcome with the all-too-familiar urge to go to the student center snack bar. She struggled with herself, recognizing she was on the verge of a binge. Her mind raced. She was very tense and desperate to try anything to stop the craving.

Terry hadn't had a particularly spiritual upbringing, but she had enrolled in a yoga class that semester and was learning about meditation and mindfulness. In a recent session, the instructor had said that meditation was an excellent way to get more in touch with one's inner guide. Because Terry hadn't had any personal experience with such a concept, she'd pushed the lecture to the back of her mind.

Now, caught in the grip of an intense craving, Terry decided to see if meditation could help her get past her relentless urge to eat. She hoped relaxing would take her mind off food so she could get through the rest of the evening in peace.

She set her book aside and closed her eyes. She began to relax by taking slow, deep breaths like they did in the yoga class. After a few minutes of calming her muscles and her mind, Terry found herself feeling much more peaceful.

While she was in this relaxed state, the instructor's discussion about the inner guide came to mind. Casting all doubt aside, she decided to apply his approach to dealing with her cravings. In a question for which she had no answer, she turned her thoughts inward and allowed herself to believe she was talking to the intuitive force her yoga instructor had talked about. She calmly asked herself, "Why do I feel so compelled to eat, even when I don't want to?"

Terry sat there in the same relaxed state for several more minutes, continuing to breathe slowly and deeply, and letting all other thoughts drift from her mind. She waited for an answer to her question, but none came to her. Slowly she opened her eyes. Much to her relief, she noted that the meditative state had taken away the immediate desire to eat, but she felt mildly disappointed that the inner guide approach hadn't worked.

No longer feeling the need to go to the student center, however, Terry picked up her book and started reading where she'd left off. She was several pages into it when suddenly, with no apparent cues, a very loud thought flashed in her mind like a bolt of lightning: "Your problems come from a poor self-image and low self-esteem."

The thought came to her so strongly that she knew instantly it was the answer to her question. She laid her book down and contemplated what she'd just heard. The more Terry thought about it, the more convinced she was that it was a message from something more than just her own thoughts. She wondered if there really was something to this inner force her teacher had talked about.

In all her years of struggling with cravings, she had never made the connection between how she regarded herself and the way she ate. At first she thought the idea that she had low self-esteem was ridiculous. She was a popular girl. She considered herself outgoing and adventurous. Her friends and professors often commented on how self-assured and confident she was.

As she sat there and tried to prove the idea wrong, however, she began to wonder if the statement might have a hint of truth. There was, she realized, a difference between being self-confident and having high self-esteem. As she considered what this voice had told her, evidence to demonstrate its point flooded into her mind. Examples of how she had unknowingly belittled herself for years came rushing to the surface as if someone had opened the gates to a dam.

She picked up a notebook and began to write. Thoughts of her childhood she had long ago suppressed were now fresh in her mind, and she wrote them down as quickly as they came to her. She had never before experienced such an awakening of memories, and she wrote nonstop, filling page after page of the notebook with increasing astonishment and exhilaration.

"That's why I tore all my old pictures out of my high school yearbooks!" she wrote as she realized that even though she'd grown to be an attractive young woman, she'd been carrying around the worn-out image of herself as a pimply faced, homely teenager with glasses.

More proof of her unrecognized poor self-image flashed into her mind. "That's why I eat too much when I have a bad hair day!" she thought.

On and on she wrote, revealing things about herself and her actions that she had never before understood. Looking at her notes, she realized she had first learned to use food to cover up bad feelings during her early teen years, a time in her life when she felt insecure about her looks and when her emotions were as confused as any normal adolescent's. She never learned to deal with those emotions in a healthy manner, and consequently, she was still carrying around a false image of herself.

Terry had a hard time getting to sleep that night. When she finally did turn out the light, it was with the notebook on her nightstand. During the night she woke up several times with more realizations about her past and of how a low self-image had contributed to her eating problems. The list grew to several pages.

The next morning as she read over the mass of hastily scribbled notes, she shook her head in amazement at the many things she had never realized were at the root of her obsession with food. Suddenly, it became obvious to her why she had never made this discovery before: she had never asked.

She realized that many times in the past she had felt the same subtle mental hints about the reason she overate, but she had ignored them. A tiny voice inside had been talking to her, but she hadn't been listening.

Terry had heard about "woman's intuition" but had never related it to the same inner guide her yoga instructor talked about. Since that day she has relied on her intuition to provide the answers to many questions, and it has never failed her.

Your own unasked questions can be answered as easily as Terry's were. Connecting with your intuition is no more difficult than talking to a friend. It requires nothing more than consciously directing your questions inward and knowing you're seeking your own internal guidance. Put all doubt aside, then direct your inquiries to the force inside you. Deliberately ask for its help.

To find out the root causes of your food cravings, you can ask general questions such as Terry asked: "Why do I feel so compelled to eat, even when I don't want to?" or "Why am I so tense?"

Once you understand why you're having a craving, you can ask for your inner guide's help in dealing with the specific emotions causing the craving by saying, for example, "I'm feeling scared and lonely this evening. I know I really don't want to eat, so please help me get past this."

Or you could say to your inner guide, "I'd like to lose a few more pounds, but I'm so bored this afternoon I'm afraid I'm going to end up eating all day. Please tell me what I can do besides eating to feel better."

Communicating with your intuition is easy. You can do it almost any time or any place. As long as you are consciously directing your words to the force inside you, you can ask your questions while driving, exercising, or cooking dinner. If you're at work and want a moment of peace, go to the restroom or some other quiet place. Close your eyes and ask your questions silently. It doesn't matter how or when you ask. The answers you're looking for are inside you. Just ask.

Learn to rely on your intuition. Get in the habit of asking yourself questions for which you have no answers. Then stay tuned in for the response. When it comes, follow the advice you hear. Once you learn how infallible your intuition is, you'll rarely find yourself in that exasperating situation of thinking, "If only I'd listened to my intuition!" You'll have far fewer regrets and will save yourself a lot of unnecessary anxiety if you make a habit of listening to the wisest voice inside you.

In order to hear the answers or the guidance when it comes to you, you have to know how to recognize the voice of your inner guide. The voice isn't always as obvious as the message that popped into Terry's mind so loudly when she asked for the cause of her cravings. It can actually be very subtle. Sometimes its presence may seem more like a feeling or a hunch.

Your inner guide's voice is different from the parent, critic, or craver voices you're so used to hearing. These voices are often much louder than the quiet messages of your intuition. Listening to these false voices will sabotage your best efforts, so it's crucial to be able to differentiate between negative messages and those of your intuition.

The key to recognizing your inner guide is knowing that its voice is always helpful and positive. It speaks only the truth. Its messages make you feel good, bringing a sense of peace. Acting on its advice fills you with peace or with positive energy and excitement. In short, if the messages you hear are negative or judgmental, they are not the voice of your intuition.

Don't worry if you don't get the answers to your questions right away. Just trust that they're on their way, then forget about them. At some time within the next few hours or days, something will send you a message that contains the advice you were looking for. It may be a voice in your head or some other external source you hadn't expected. You may have temporarily forgotten you asked the question, but because you so deliberately asked, you'll recognize the answer when it comes to you, no matter how it's delivered.

Each time you get a response to a question you asked your inner guide, you'll feel like you've made an amazing discovery. You'll begin to trust that your intuition is a real force you haven't been taking advantage of. You'll become convinced of its helpfulness and you'll realize it will never let you down.

If you've spent years bemoaning the fact that you have a problem dealing with food, but have never taken the time to uncover the reasons, the following exercise will provide you starting points with which to address your inner guide.

Exercise: Inner Guide

Use the space below to list questions that you can direct to your inner guide. Leave room after each one. Later, when you ask them at an appropriate time, you can record the answers as they come to you. It can be especially interesting to note the manner in which you become aware of the answers.

Questions:

Answers Received:

By tuning in to and listening to your intuition, you will not only feel more at peace, you'll develop a much closer relationship with yourself (or more accurately, with your *Self*). You will experience a sense of connectedness not only with yourself, but with those around you as you realize that everyone has this same powerful inner source.

When you trust that your inner guide exists and tap into its resources, your battle with cravings will be infinitely easier. This source will guide you to greater awareness than you ever thought possible. Just think, you no longer have to do all the work! With the help of this inner guide, you won't have to deal with your emotions and anxiety by yourself. If you're willing to simply believe that this guiding force will send you the messages you need to deal with feelings and conquer cravings, you're ready to take step three and *listen* to your intuition.

Sometimes it's hard to trust advice when it comes from within. We'd be much more confident if the advice came from some known expert such as a therapist or teacher. Until you've had several wake-up calls from your inner advisor, simply try to throw all apprehension aside.

Once you've experienced how intuition can work for you, any doubts you have will be replaced with certainty. There will be no question that it is a true force that can be called upon for direction.

Just as airplane passengers turn control of the plane over to the pilot, you can turn your eating over to your intuition by trusting that it will tell you when to eat and what to eat. It will answer your most troubling questions. It will show you how to overcome your cravings. All you have to do is relax and listen.

12
Let Your Inner Guide Handle It

Many people who have a problem with food find it hard to relax. They like to control things, especially themselves. Just as they try to control their actions, they also try to control everything that goes into their mouths. They let their parental voices dominate and tell themselves what they should or shouldn't eat.

Are you constantly struggling to control your actions? Do you think of some foods as bad? Are there others that are on your personal forbidden foods list? Do you feel like a failure if, heaven forbid, you eat something that's not good for you? If so, you're controlling too much and making yourself miserable. It's time to lighten up and let your inner guide handle it.

All the symptoms of a craving point to your inner conflict: knots in your stomach, restricted or rapid breathing, tense muscles, and maybe even a sense of heaviness or depression. Think back to the subconscious conversations you read between a typical craver and the voice of her cravings. What one thing was always present? Tension.

Your intuition doesn't work that way. It doesn't talk in shoulds or shouldn'ts. It tells it like it is. If you find yourself struggling not to eat, if you find yourself fighting off a craving, that is a prime indicator that you are *not* listening to your intuition.

What are you struggling against? You're struggling against your intuition. It knows best. It's trying to tell you what to do, but if you're struggling with a craving, you're resisting it.

Think about what happens if your doctor tells you to exercise three times a week for your health, but you decide not to take the advice. There you are, sitting comfortably on your couch, when you see a jogger pass by your window. How do you feel? You feel guilty. And what happens? You tense up, knowing you should be out there exercising. You feel bad because you're not following the advice of the experts and doing what's good for you.

The same thing happens when you don't listen to your own built-in expert. Your inner guide knows what's best for you in every situation. It constantly sends you guidance, but you may not be listening. Or you may be listening, but you may not want to comply with what you hear.

If thoughts of eating are causing you conflict, that's the first sign that you're going against your intuition. Pay attention to your body's signals. When you become aware that you're not comfortable, content, or relaxed, realize that you're struggling with your *Self*. When one voice in your head is telling you to eat while another is telling you not to, it's no wonder you're tense.

If you take a moment to quiet your controlling voices, you'll hear your intuition telling you when and what to eat. You can find instant relief from the conflict by releasing your need to control and giving that responsibility to your inner guide. Turn your struggle over to it. Let your intuition take control of what you eat.

There's no need for willpower. There's no need for self- discipline. By taking step three and listening to your intuition, you no longer have to worry about controlling what you eat.

The human mind is a funny thing. The more you try to suppress, resist, or deny something, the more you think about it. If you tell yourself you won't eat chocolate anymore, chances are you'll obsess all day about biting into a candy bar, simply because you're attracted to what you can't have.

By allowing yourself to eat anything you want, you ensure that the foods you crave most often will lose their attraction. This may be a hard concept to accept, but when you couple it with step three, it's not so strange. After giving yourself permission to eat whatever you like in any amount, you simply need to listen for your intuition to guide you. If you feel anxious about eating something, that's the sign that you're going against your intuition. So don't do it! It's that simple.

If, on the other hand, it feels okay to eat whatever you want, even if it's a double-decker fudge brownie sundae, then go ahead. If you're aware of your body's signals, and there's no tension, you have permission. There's a lot to be learned from the phrase, "If it feels good, do it!"

You may go a little crazy at first, eating what you consider too much or wrong, but remember, there are no good foods or bad foods anymore. You've given yourself permission to eat anything. And if you truly listen to your intuition, once you get over the initial euphoria of being allowed to eat at will, it won't be long before you settle down and eat only what your body needs or can handle at the moment.

If you eat a little much, that's okay because your intuition will tell you how to make up for it, either by encouraging you to exercise or letting you know when you need to eat less. Stop worrying and just listen to your body.

If the concept of allowing yourself to eat dessert every day is just too hard to accept, you can always ask for guidance, right? Before you take that first bite of chocolate cake, ask your inner guide, "How is cake for dessert tonight?" If it feels right, that's your intuition giving you the green light. If you get the definite feeling that Jello would be a better idea, follow your intuition and skip the cake.

Along with giving yourself permission to eat, there's also tremendous power in giving yourself permission *not* to eat something. Think about the last time you were out shopping and got a craving for something really sinful. Your intuition might have been telling you that you didn't need anything, but you went ahead and bought something to eat anyway.

There you were, walking around the mall with a giant gourmet chocolate chip cookie or a double scoop of ice cream. You took that first luscious bite, but were overcome with guilt. Why? Because your intuition was trying to tell you the snack wasn't the right thing to indulge in at the moment, but you were fighting it.

So, take back your personal power. The next time you find yourself in the same type of situation, listen to your intuition right then and there and throw out what remains of your little indulgence. Okay, so you may have just blown a dollar or two, but isn't peace of mind worth at least that much to you? Give yourself permission to not eat what's in your hand, and experience the power of following your inner guide.

- Throw the cookie in the trash can!
- Toss a half-eaten doughnut out your car window at 65 miles per hour. The birds will eat it.
- Leave two bites of spaghetti on your dinner plate.
- Let somebody else eat that last potato chip!

Listen to your intuition and do whatever feels right. Give yourself permission to eat if it feels good, or give yourself permission not to eat if doing so would make you feel bad.

Trying to stay in control hasn't worked. It has only caused you conflict and guilt, so give it up. Turn over the compulsion to eat to your inner guide. Tell your Self, "I can't handle this right now. I don't want to fight. You take care of it."

Then stop struggling and let your inner guide do the work for you.

13

Meditation

Hopefully, by now you're anxious to begin accessing the helpful guidance that's inside you. In addition to simply asking questions and listening to the answers, there's another easy way to get in touch with your intuition. Just like in Terry's story, you can communicate with your inner guide while meditating. This highly relaxed state helps quiet your mind, making it easier to hear any answers that are readily available.

In recent years meditation has become identified mainly with the New Age movement. Mention meditation and visions of people sitting cross-legged on the floor chanting mantras come to mind. There is really nothing strange about meditation, however. Even some of the most conservative, right-brained people engage in quiet reflection from time to time.

So what exactly is meditation? In the strictest definition of the word, meditation is nothing more than deep relaxation with a still mind. It is a quiet period when you slow the thoughts running around your brain, tune in to your Self. and listen. For those who are trying to overcome cravings by getting more in touch with their thoughts and feelings, this type of self-therapy can work wonders.

Many people believe meditation involves completely emptying the brain of all thoughts. As you've already discovered, it's impossible to do this. Instead of blocking your thoughts, meditation only requires that you quiet your body and mind. It's a deliberate slowing down of all physical and mental activity.

Our lives are so busy that we rarely take time to just listen. When you put your hectic life on hold for just a few minutes a day, you give yourself the opportunity to discover that the qualities you so fervently search for outside yourself actually originate inside you.

Some people try meditating a few times and give up when nothing miraculous happens. They mistakenly think they're doing it wrong. There is no right or wrong way to meditate. There are no hard-and-fast rules to follow, just a few basic guidelines.

You can meditate for one minute or one hour. You can play soft music in the background or relax in total silence. You can chant one-syllable words or not make a sound. You can visualize a pleasant scene or focus on nothing at all. You can communicate with your higher power or you can simply listen for whatever thoughts come to mind.

Meditation in its most basic form is quite easy. All you have to do is follow these fundamental steps:

1. Find a few minutes to devote to your peace of mind.
2. Choose a quiet place where you won't be interrupted.
3. Get comfortable.
4. Relax your body from head to toe.
5. Quiet your mind.
6. Listen, pray, or ponder for as long as you'd like.
7. Open your eyes and return to what you were doing, enjoying the peaceful feelings you've created.

That's what meditation is all about: finding the love, joy, and peace within you.

These three basic ingredients are what all of us need for a happy life, and all can be achieved through the simple process of connecting with yourself on a regular basis. Changing your focus from looking out to looking within is a part of your recovery from your preoccupation with food. Meditation helps you by increasing your awareness of your thoughts and how you direct them. It helps you become more in tune with how your body reacts to what goes on in your mind. As an added bonus, this deliberate form of relaxation also provides a non-addictive, chemical-free method to reduce stress, which can be a major craving trigger.

While stress may be a contributor to your cravings, it's also a necessary part of life. Stress is what gets you going and keeps you out of danger. There is, however, good stress and bad stress. The pressure of trying to do too much, too quickly, with too few resources is the kind that leads to high blood pressure, ulcers, smoking, drinking, and of course, overeating.

People who are under too much stress are more likely to suffer from depression. They get irritable and snappy, and have trouble handling normally routine tasks. They find it hard to relax, even when there's a lull in their hectic lives, and often have aches and pains associated with muscular tension.

Like negative emotions, stress can be uncomfortable to deal with. You can try to fight it, you can shove it down with food, or you can find a healthier way to deal with it. That's where meditation comes in. Meditation is the craver's answer to stress-related eating. It's impossible to meditate without first passing into a very relaxed state, since the first few minutes are spent quieting the mind and relaxing the body. This is the exact prescription for dealing with the stress that can bring on a craving.

You can't meditate all day, however, so between meditations you should strive to achieve balance in your life. Balance the time you work with the time you devote to your family and yourself. If you're spending too much time on the job or doing other chores, take a look at your priorities. See how you can find some way to bring more joy into your life. If free time is at a minimum, how can you make your work more fun?

Stress is a sign that your life is out of balance. Strive for harmony between your physical, mental, and spiritual selves. Are you exercising your muscles or sitting around all day? Are you burned out because your work is mentally taxing? Do you take time to connect with your inner guide?

Meditation can help level things out. On the physical side, it helps relax your tense muscles. On the mental side, it eases the strain your mind is under by quieting it, if only for a few minutes.

Best of all, on the spiritual side, meditation is an excellent way to connect with your intuition. The source of wisdom inside you is constantly speaking to you, but it's often hard to hear its voice through the crowd of other voices buzzing in your head. In meditation, those many voices are quieted, and your intuition can finally be heard. Even if you don't actually hear its wise advice, in this peaceful state you can easily access your subconscious mind and memories.

Exercise: Meditation

The following is a sample meditation you can use to ease your stress and connect with your inner guide. To get the greatest benefit, read it aloud into a tape recorder. Review it several times before actually recording it so you get a feel for how slowly you need to speak and how long you should pause between phrases.

For a more calming effect, play soft music in the background while you're recording. Speak in a quiet, soothing voice. This will be your own private tape, so don't worry about how you sound.

Replaying your recording through a cassette deck works fine, but the best way to meditate while using a tape of your voice or other music is with headphones. This way you'll block out distracting noises and enter your own private world, if only for a few minutes a day.

Most record stores or gift shops sell special tapes with mood music that's perfect for accompanying your meditations. The best include repetitive, soothing sounds such as waves lapping against the seashore or the soft tones of wind chimes.

Sit on the floor or in a comfortable chair. Loosen any tight clothing. Uncross your legs. Start your tape player, then rest your hands lightly on your thighs, palms up or down, whichever is most natural for you. Close your eyes and follow the instructions from your tape.

One final note before you get started: It's best not to lie down while meditating since you may fall asleep if you get too cozy. Meditation is such a relaxing activity that this could happen even if you sit up straight. If you do catch yourself napping, either try again immediately or have a go at it later. Be persistent. The tendency to fall asleep eventually disappears.

Now that you're ready, start recording. (Do not record the words in parentheses.)

With your eyes closed, begin to relax. Start with a deep, cleansing breath . . . breathe in slowly. . . (long pause). . . now exhale. . . Again, breathe in deeply through your mouth... (long pause). . . breathe out. . . . As you exhale, imagine all the tension in your body flowing out with your breath. One more time, breathe in... and out, feeling the stress leaving your body.

Continue to relax by releasing the tension from each part of your body. Start with your toes and your feet. Imagine they're resting on a soft pillow. They have no tension at all. Move up to your calves. Focus on the muscles and allow them to relax. Move up past your knees to your thighs. Mentally shake out all the tension that has built up in your legs.

Focus your attention on your hips and your abdominal area. move up to your chest . . . relax your entire torso. You're feeling calm and peaceful as your anxiety slips away. Now focus on your hands. They feel heavy as they rest on your legs. If you were to lift your arm now, it would fall like a heavy weight. Mentally move up through your arms, relaxing your forearms. . . now your biceps and triceps.... Continue breathing slowly and deeply. . . you're so relaxed.

Now move into the shoulder area. You have a lot of tension here. . . let it flow through you. . . your shoulders and back are completely relaxed. Release all the stress that remains in this area . . . relax your neck. .

Breathing ever more slowly. . . focus now on your head and face. The rest of your body is free of tension. Let all the muscles in your face go slack. Relax your forehead. . . your eyelids. . . your cheeks... your lips are completely soft... the muscles around your mouth have no tension. . .

Now relax your mind. . . . . As thoughts come to you, allow them to flow through you. Your breathing is getting slower and deeper. You are more and more relaxed with every breath. Imagine that a river of warmth begins to flow through you. It starts at the top of your head... (pause). . . imagine it flowing into your body. . . flowing slowly down through all parts of you.

As the warmth flows through you, it fills you with a sense of peace. Feel the warmth as it flows through your arms, moving slowly until it fills each finger. The warmth spreads through your chest. . . into your stomach, surrounding your internal organs, warming all of you.... It continues down through your legs.

Imagine that as the warmth flows through you that it carries off every remaining bit of tension in your body. All your stress is flowing on this current of warmth. As the stream reaches your toes, you allow the stress to flow completely out of your body... (pause)... your entire body is now filled with warmth..

Now imagine the warmth surrounding your body and filling the room. It's as if you are in a soft cocoon. You feel safe, comforted, and loved. This warmth is coming from somewhere above you. Allow yourself to mentally travel up the stream of warmth. You lift your face as you travel higher, growing ever more comfortable and relaxed the higher you go.

As you approach the source of the warmth, you find yourself entering a large space. What do you see in this warm room? (Pause.) This is where you'll connect with *your inner guide. What does it look like? (Pause.) Take a few moments to look around and get acquainted. (Long pause.)*

When you are ready to meet your inner guide, ask it to appear. (Long pause.) As you become aware of the presence of your guide, greet your guide and thank it for being there. How does your guide look? Is it a man or a woman? Does it have human characteristics or is it formless? Ask your guide what it would like to be called and see if a name comes to you. (Long pause.)

Your guide is here in this space to help you. Use this time to ask it for the answer to any question that has been troubling you. (Long pause.) Stay in this place as long as you like. Be receptive to any answers your guide may send you. If no answers come to you right away, remain relaxed, knowing that you will get a reply at some time in the near future. (Long pause.)

Feel the love and warmth that surround you in this inviting place. When you are ready to leave, say good-bye to your guide.

Slowly return to your starting point. Begin to notice where you are... become aware of your body... open your eyes and return to full consciousness...

Take a few minutes to enjoy this feeling of total peace. (end of recording)

And there you have it. You may have noticed that the process of relaxing during the first few minutes of a meditation is just like that used by a hypnotist. Your goal should be to reach a state of total relaxation. This is the type of near-hypnotic state you should aim for.

When you finish this meditation, you may feel as if you've just had a good night's sleep. You'll be completely relaxed, but at the same time, you'll feel refreshed and energized. You may even have a smile on your face. Any stress you had before you meditated will be greatly reduced or even completely gone. If you were meditating in response to a craving, the urge to eat will have disappeared.

This scenario is just one example of the way you can direct your thoughts while meditating. You can create any scene that makes you feel peaceful. Imagine yourself walking down a quiet path in the woods or sitting on a majestic mountaintop. You don't have to picture anything. You may opt instead to concentrate on the part of your body where you imagine your inner spirit resides and direct your thoughts and questions there. Remember, there is no wrong or right way to meditate. Follow the previous guidelines and you'll be fine.

After you've experienced the peace and pleasure that come from meditating, you may become hooked. Your meditation time will become a gift you give yourself every day. It will become a healthy escape from a busy, stressful day.

Nothing will convince you more of the benefits of meditation than trying it for yourself. As often as you need to, look for ten to twenty minutes when you can be alone. If you share your home, you may need to ask your family or friends for their cooperation to allow you these few minutes of peace. If they're not used to this new side of you, explain to them what meditation is about and why you're doing it. Who knows? They may even get interested enough to try it themselves.

As with many new ventures, you may start off with enthusiasm, devoting twenty minutes a day to meditation. But over time, you may find you're giving less and less time to yourself. If this happens, remember that meditation is about balance. It is meant to ease your stress, not add to it. Use it as needed, and add it to the many tools you now have available to overcome your cravings.

Part IV
Treat Yourself Lovingly

14

Be Your Own Best Friend

By learning to follow the first three steps in the HALT process, you already have a powerful arsenal at your disposal for fighting off cravings. After all the hard work, however, you may be feeling a little battle weary at this point.

All good military leaders know that in order to have a capable fighting force, they have to take care of their people. Their soldiers need good, healthy food and a warm, dry place to sleep in order to be ready for battle. When they're tired, they need rest. When morale is low, a little pep talk and encouragement can work wonders.

On the other side of the coin, soldiers need to know they're needed and that their efforts are doing some good. They want to be treated with respect. If they're treated well, they'll give everything they've got. This is a fundamental leadership concept, and it works as well in fighting cravings as it does on the battlefield.

If you are not treating yourself kindly, appreciatively, and with respect, you are undermining all your good efforts. To eliminate your cravings, you have to eliminate self-defeating behaviors that work against your ultimate victory. The fourth and final step in the HALT process asks you to stop sabotaging your success and *treat* yourself lovingly.

From one moment to the next, how good are you to yourself? You may be treating yourself poorly on a routine basis and not even know it. Starting with the way you talk to yourself, take a look and see if you are subconsciously undermining your efforts to improve your eating habits. You can do this with the following short exercise designed to examine your self-talk in a variety of situations. Your answers may surprise and enlighten you.

Exercise: Self-Talk

Choose the phrase you would most likely say to yourself in the following scenarios. Be as honest as you can, even if your intuition tells you what the preferred answer is. (See . . . you can rely on your intuition for any number of things.)

1. You accidentally spill a glass of milk.
a. What a klutz! I am so darned clumsy!
b. What a mess! At least the glass didn't break.

2. You try on a pair of pants that are somewhat snug.
a. These pants look awful. I am so fat!
b. Wow. I don't like the cut of these pants at all. I'd better pick a style that's more flattering to my figure.

3. You eat two servings of birthday cake at your own party.
a. I'm such a pig. No wonder I can't lose weight.
b. It's a good thing birthdays come around only once a year. Tomorrow I'll have to cut back.

4. You are taking a class, and when called upon, you give a wrong answer.
a. I'm so stupid! Everyone must think I'm an idiot.
b. That was embarrassing. Oh well, looks like nobody else knew the answer either.

5. You thought you'd gotten rid of your cravings for good, but one hits you unexpectedly after a long string of successes.
a. Oh, no, here I go again! I'm a failure. I'll never change.
b. Hmm. I must not be doing something right. I'd better go back over what I've learned and try again.

It should be obvious that if you chose the first answer to any of the scenarios, your self-talk is on the harsh side. Unfortunately, most people are more likely to choose self-talk *a* rather than *b* when talking to themselves. Their immediate reaction to most situations is to put themselves down. The sad thing is, they would never talk that way to their best friend.

Could you imagine telling a friend, "You are so dumb," or "You sure look fat today"? One thing's sure, they wouldn't be your friends for long if that's the way you talked to them. So why do you use such unkind, judgmental words on yourself?

If your best friend heard you referring to yourself using any of the first group of sentences in the exercise, she'd probably jump to your defense immediately, telling you to go easy on yourself. She'd give you encouragement rather than criticize you. She'd downplay or even overlook your faults rather than focusing on them. In short, she'd treat you lovingly.

Admit it. You can be your own worst critic. When what you really want is to be loved and accepted by those around you, often you don't afford yourself the same kind of treatment and respect. Being treated lovingly starts with you—with the way you view yourself, talk to yourself, and take care of yourself.

Just like negative thoughts, negative self-talk may be aggravating your cravings. Learn to listen to the way you talk to yourself. Constantly berating yourself only adds to your negative feelings by lowering your self-esteem. That's the last thing you need when one of your goals is to raise your self-esteem. You need to make your self-talk work for you, not against you.

Even something so seemingly insignificant as how you address yourself in your inner conversations can make a big difference in how you feel. For example, what name do you habitually use when talking to yourself? Is it what your parents called you when they were pleased with you or is it the name they used when they were angry? If your parents were like most, you could always tell by the way they said your name if you were in trouble, couldn't you? Little "Debbie" suddenly became "Deborah" or "Eddie" became "Edward."

Try addressing yourself in your self-talk with a favorite nickname, even if you would never introduce yourself to other adults that way. Really. Try it right now. Without speaking out loud, say to yourself, "Hey, (using your nickname), you're okay by me."

How does that make you feel? Just as certain scents evoke pleasant memories, a special name can be linked to good feelings, too, and with this one simple technique you can bring back those pleasant feelings at will.

Treating yourself lovingly begins with talking to yourself lovingly. Be kind, sympathetic, supportive, encouraging, and forgiving. Remember, you're addressing a friend. Use endearing terms with yourself. Refuse to be judgmental. Be accepting of your faults. Be both coach and cheerleader. You should be your biggest fan.

While you're at it, treat yourself the way you wish others would treat you. We all want to be loved and nurtured, but too often we wait for others to do the nurturing for us. We talk about giving ourselves a pat on the back for our good deeds, but how often do we actually do it? Literally. Try patting yourself on the back or arm while you say a loving, encouraging phrase (and don't forget to use your favorite name). Better yet, put your hand on your cheek and say it. These things are probably best done in private, but they are tremendous ways of showing yourself how important you are.

When you were little, what did you do with your best friend? Did you enjoy playing together? Did you have fun and act silly? Grown-ups are so serious. Sometimes we carry the weight of the world on our shoulders. You may be so preoccupied with your cravings and other problems that you no longer allow yourself the luxury of temporarily putting your worries aside and playing.

Inside you is the same little kid from your childhood days. Parts of you have grown up, but there's still a child who needs to feel loved, who craves attention, and who wants to be free to have fun.

The little child in you also needs to feel safe and protected. She wants to be forgiven for her behavior when she didn't know any other way to act. She needs to be listened to and to know that you care about her. Sometimes, she just wants to cry and be held and comforted.

These childhood needs and emotions don't go away as you grow up. Listen to the child voices inside you and attend to those needs. If you ignore this part of you, the little child will act up, just like kids are prone to do. If you don't listen to the little kid in you and treat her lovingly, her needs will be manifested in other ways, many times as the desire to eat.

Just as using affirmations and positive thoughts will change your belief system, consistently using kind self-talk and appealing to the child you used to be will improve the way you feel about yourself. Even if you've spent your whole life putting yourself down, or listening to others do it for you, by consciously supporting and nurturing yourself through loving inner conversations and actions, you will create a happier, more confident person who has no need for cravings.

Stuffing yourself with food is not a loving way to treat yourself. Think about how you feel after overeating. Mentally, you feel guilty and depressed. Physically, your stomach hurts, and you may be shaky, hyperactive, or drowsy, depending on how your body reacts to too much food.

When you realize that the power to create your own happiness lies within, you won't look to food to do it for you. When you're kind to yourself, you automatically create thoughts that make you feel good, and food loses its importance.

In the past, you acted on your cravings by eating. This was an unhealthy response, bringing only temporary relief. But you didn't know how else to react. Now you know better. Applying all the strategies you've learned so far is a much more loving way to deal with your food obsession.

You now know how to turn your thoughts around by listening to your mental conversations. You've practiced carrying on an objective dialogue with your counselor. You're learning how to listen to your intuition to help you deal with your feelings. When you recognize that you can't get food off your mind because you're feeling down, you've learned you can rely on your intuition to tell you what would feel better than eating.

Your inner guide is an excellent source of advice on positive alternatives to eating. Just ask. Often the guidance you receive results in activities that will lift your spirits. After all, there aren't many activities that would make you feel *worse* than the way you feel after giving in to a craving.

Taking action and doing something healthy and fun rather than giving in to a binge is something positive you can do to treat yourself well. By doing so, you're getting in the habit of seeking new and creative ways of taking care of yourself, rather than falling into the same old self-destructive habits.

There are all kinds of short-term remedies to help you get past the crucial few minutes when a craving is at its strongest point. You've probably seen lists of these craving side-trackers in women's magazines. They're designed to get your mind off your stomach and onto something more healthy than overeating. These kinds of suggestions are best for cravings that hit when you're feeling bored or restless. They work because they help you find more productive ways to direct your energy than sitting alone and stuffing yourself with food.

The following methods to treat yourself lovingly are representative of these ever-popular instant craving-stopper lists. Rather than eating, they recommend you overcome your cravings by doing some of the following:

1. Wait twenty minutes or more until the desire to eat disappears on its own.

This method of stopping a craving works because whatever negative thought or emotion triggered the craving in the first place is either forgotten or replaced with another thought while the time passes. For people who aren't listening to their thoughts, however, this can be a difficult and somewhat risky way to overcome cravings. The time when your cravings are strongest is usually when you feel your most vulnerable, and it's far too easy to give in to the craving before twenty minutes are up. Unless, of course, you remember to remain aware of what's going on in your mind and call a HALT. If you use those twenty minutes to hear your thoughts and feel the emotions they cause, perhaps even carrying on a conscious mental dialogue with your counselor voice, you'll be making the best possible use of your time. Don't just put in time waiting for the cravings to go away on their own. Put in the necessary effort and make time work to your advantage.

2. Exercise.

Working out is an excellent way to get your mind off food and reduce stress. Of course, this option may not be practical or advisable in the middle of a business meeting or while sitting in rush-hour traffic. If, however, your craving hits while you're sitting around watching TV or reading, treat yourself to a brisk walk, jog, bike ride, or other activity that gets your blood pumping. Yes, it takes real motivation to get up off the couch and do something physical, but if you give yourself a pep talk and get moving instead of giving in to your cravings, you'll be much more satisfied and energized within the hour than if you'd sat there and eaten a pint of ice cream.

3. Listen to music.

Music is magical. It soothes, it energizes, it can change your attitude in an instant. Have a variety of music on hand for every mood, so that when a craving hits and you've identified what feelings triggered it, you can pop in just the right tunes to improve your mood. Put on a pair of headphones or blast your stereo. Move to the beat. Sing out loud. Really get into it! Whether it's rock and roll or a piano concerto, let the healing sounds of music carry you beyond your craving.

4. Go shopping.

This can be a somewhat costly alternative to overeating, but some people find great solace in treating themselves to a shopping spree. It's all part of treating yourself lovingly. Of course, if seeing and smelling food in a mall food court is a major craving trigger for you, you may want to choose your destination carefully.

5. Get a manicure.

There's a very good reason why this craving remedy works: you won't be able to touch food for at least half an hour until your nails dry! All kidding aside, this tip is included simply to show that there are any number of ways to give yourself a treat other than with food.

6. Call a friend to chat.

You can turn to your inner guide any time you need help getting through a craving. You can also call in your counselor and talk yourself through it. There's nothing like sharing your thoughts and feelings with a friend, however, to provide you with a loving sanity check at those times when you're feeling most vulnerable.

Members of twelve-step programs know very well the value of support from others who are dealing with the same problem and working toward the same goals. If you have a friend you trust enough to confide in about your new undertaking to conquer your cravings, enlist her support to help you when the road gets bumpy. Ask permission to give her a call when you're fighting the urge to raid the refrigerator. Tell her what you're going through and let her know how to help you. Knowing there's someone else who cares and is rooting for you can be very comforting. She can even remind you to call a HALT if you get too caught up in your craving to remember to do so yourself.

So what happens if your craving confidant isn't available? Call anyone. You don't have to pour out your problems—just have a friendly conversation with another human being and catch up on what's new. Rid yourself of boredom, loneliness, and frustration and get through your craving by connecting with another human being.

7. Write a letter.

This craving-stopper goes hand in hand with the previous one. Pick up a pen and paper or sit down at your word processor. Even though you're not talking in person, writing to a friend or family member gives you a positive outlet for your emotions.

And how about one more? The previous examples showed you how to make yourself feel better by chatting with a friend or writing a letter. This was all about connecting with another human being. If you're fighting the urge to overeat and don't know what to do to feel better, why not grab (literally) your spouse or significant other and enjoy yourselves. Surprise them. You don't have to let them know they're a substitute for a jelly doughnut! You'll have a much more enjoyable time than sitting by yourself eating, and you'll relieve some stress at the same time.

These types of activities really are effective ways to stop a craving at any given moment. While on the surface they seem simply to be ways of avoiding your problems, they do the job by creating positive feelings. They improve your mood and help you turn negative emotions into positive ones. They show your subconscious you care enough to take care of yourself.

The problem with these solutions, however, is that they are short-term fixes. If your intuition tells you that rather than eating, you should go for a walk in the woods, by all means, do so. For a more lasting remedy, however, the fourth step also asks that you make a concerted effort to change the way you treat yourself every minute of the day.

15

Long-Term Loving Strategies

In the last chapter you learned how to treat yourself lovingly by being your own best friend. This included a few fast-acting techniques for getting past your cravings when they hit. You'll be happy to know that the fourth step also includes some things you can do for yourself that will actually help ward off cravings *before* they hit.

Some of these are mental strategies, falling into the category of psychological operations, which add extra power to your arsenal of craving-fighters. The others require you to take deliberate action and do loving things for your body. All of them work because they help eliminate the craving-causers you now recognize: false or incorrect thoughts and beliefs, negative feelings, unmet needs, low self-esteem, and the need to control.

Long-Term Strategy One: Throw away your bathroom scales

You may be thinking, "What? Are you kidding? I could never do that! How will I know how much I weigh if I don't step on my scales every day?"

The answer to that is: what difference does it make? The number on a scale is a relative figure. One person who weighs 120 pounds could look completely different from another who weighs exactly the same. While you can certainly use scales to monitor whether your weight is going up or down, what really matters is how you look in the mirror and how your clothes fit. Use your clothing to tell you if you need to cut back on what you eat. Check your naked body in the mirror to see if your weight is where you want it to be. Learn to rely on your intuition and other senses such as sight and touch, rather than an arbitrary number.

If throwing out your scales strikes terror in your heart, you are addicted to them. Like most scale addicts, your daily routine probably goes something like this:

- You get on the scales at least once a day.
- You weigh yourself first thing in the morning, before you eat or drink anything, making sure you're completely naked so you're at your absolute lightest.
- If you don't like the weight you see, you get off the scales and get back on. You may even bounce up and down a lit- tie to see if the number changes.
- If your weight has gone down, you're ecstatic and guaranteed to have a good day.
- If your weight has gone up, your day is already a complete loss and your cravings are likely to begin any minute.

Allowing your weight to set your mood for the day sets you up for failure. Your weight can easily fluctuate by several pounds a day depending on such factors as hormones, salt intake, or how much you drank the night before. A gain of a pound or two can be temporary, but if you let what the scale tells you determine how you feel, how you interpret that number can lead to a day of bingeing.

If weighing yourself only serves to make you miserable, don't do it. Get rid of those scales. And don't just put them in the back of the closet. You'll be digging them out before you know it.

If you have trouble throwing your scales in the trash, ask yourself why you're afraid of being without them. It may be that you're still not ready to trust yourself completely. That's okay for now. Make a note that this is an issue you may want to work on.

Once you make the break from your scales, if you simply can't stand not knowing what your weight is, save your weigh- ins for periodic medical checkups or visits to the gym. Just don't get hung up on the numbers. Learn to rely on yourself rather than letting an inanimate object set your mood for the day.

Long-Term Strategy Two: Don't diet

Regularly eating in response to anything other than hunger can easily lead to unwanted weight gain. Not everyone who suffers from food cravings is overweight, but if you've been ignoring your intuition and taking in more calories than your metabolism can burn off, you may have a weight problem. If your problem with cravings has indeed led you to be unhappy with your body size, chances are you're no stranger to dieting.

Veteran dieters know that in the wake of successful weight loss, you can feel like you're on top of the world. All your friends compliment you on the way you look. You have a new wardrobe and have moved your fat clothes into the back of the closet. You feel sexy and desirable. This is all terrific incentive to keep those pounds off.

So why is it that sooner or later you end up pulling out those pre-diet pants and putting your new wardrobe in storage instead? And why didn't you throw away those old, bigger clothes in the first place?

Because diets don't work.

Okay, sure, it is possible to lose weight by dieting. Everyone knows someone who has slimmed down by following the latest program. The ladies in magazine and TV ads who show off their "before-and-after" pictures have obviously succeeded. But the question is: how many of those dieters lose the weight and keep it off? What do those women look like a year later? How long was it until they regained all the weight they lost and ended up back on the diet treadmill again? If you've been on more than one diet in your lifetime, you know the lost weight has a way of creeping back.

That's because diets set you up for failure. In the back of your dieting mind, you know that the way you're eating is only temporary. The whole time you're cutting back, you're looking forward to when the diet's over. Pizza and desserts are the rewards that are waiting if you can just be "good" for a few more weeks.

Because of the mentality that diets are a temporary measure, dieters make the mistake of seeing their changes in eating habits as merely a means to an end. A diet is something you go on then get off when the desired goal has been reached. When the days of eating celery sticks and cucumbers are over, the standard reaction to all that perceived deprivation is to go right back to your old, pre-diet ways because the eating habits you were following while on the diet did not become habits at all.

If you ate packaged diet food, you're even more disadvantaged because you didn't prepare your own food. Everything was done for you. Is that realistic? Did you learn anything about shopping for and preparing healthy meals? What happens when the boxes run out and you're faced with cooking for yourself again?

If, while you're on a diet, you are only focusing on the singular goal of losing weight, your success will be short-lived. Unless you attack the inner problems that led you to overeat by diligently working the four steps in the HALT process, you're fighting a losing battle from the start.

Dieting has a nasty way of aggravating your cravings because it usually involves depriving you of your favorite foods. After all, *diet* and *deprivation* are only a few pages apart in the dictionary. Knowing that a diet will only last a fixed period of time, motivated dieters can put their willpower into high gear and struggle through the cravings long enough to see positive results.

If you're able to fight off the urge to indulge until you get down to your target weight, you may even convince yourself that you've dieted for the last time. Unfortunately, if you've been on more than one diet, you've already proven to yourself that there rarely is a last time.

Every time you find your weight has crept back up, you're forced to admit that the last attempt wasn't the final one after all. Despite your good intentions, the next time you go on a diet there will always be a nagging doubt that any weight you lose this time around may be regained just like before. How depressing.

Diets aren't merely unkind to your psyche; they mess with your body's internal thermostat. As soon as you start dieting, your body notices there's not as much fuel coming in as it's used to. To compensate for this change and protect itself against starvation, the body immediately slows down its metabolism. It tries to conserve energy in case this food drought continues.

A higher metabolism burns more calories. Therefore, when you drastically reduce your intake, your body's natural reaction is to slow down and burn fewer calories. So, while you're going to all that trouble and depriving yourself of your favorite foods, your body is not even burning off any extra fat.

After one or more low-calorie diets, your body begins to work harder and harder to adjust to the fluctuating calories you're feeding it. Yo-yo dieting, the repetitive cycle of going on a diet, regaining what you lost, then dieting again, can actually make you gain weight.

That's because the body doesn't like all this change. It has a certain weight it thinks it should maintain, called your *set point*. This is largely a hereditary factor, but it's also determined by your metabolism. On a reduced-calorie diet, your body slows down its metabolism to try and maintain the higher weight it's used to. In order to lose weight, you have to get beyond your set point and actually create a lower one.

Couch potatoes would rather not hear this, but there is really only one way to increase your metabolism and lower your set point: by exercising regularly and sticking to a reasonable eating plan. The safest, most effective way to do this is by making slow, permanent lifestyle changes you can live with. In doing so, you'll also be helping to eradicate your cravings. Why? Because eating right and exercising are two of the best ways to treat yourself lovingly.

We're surrounded by advertisements that tell us we can "lose ten pounds in ten days" or "fit into a swimsuit by summer." Human beings are impatient by nature. When it comes to getting into shape, we want to change our bodies instantly, either by crash dieting or exercising to excess. If you're not happy with the way your body looks, chances are it didn't get that way overnight. The sad truth is, it's physically impossible to change it back overnight, either—at least, not if you want it to stay that way.

Just like working with affirmations and following all the other craving-stoppers in the HALT process, ending the yo-yo diet syndrome and replacing it with long-term, permanent eating and exercise habits that fit your lifestyle takes hard work. The effort you put into it, however, will pay off in great rewards as your new habits make you feel great, physically and mentally.

Exercise will be discussed in the next section. As for diets, decide today if you're ready to give them up forever. If so, start now to make small dietary changes you can comfortably live with for the rest of your life. Figure out what's been contributing to your weight gain and make adjustments. Pay attention to how much you eat in a day. Get in the habit of reading nutrition labels and determining what percentage of the food you eat come from fat.

Take time to find out what constitutes a balanced diet and aim to eat healthier meals. Read books such as *Fight Fat and Win* by Elaine Moquette-Magee for tips on how to lower the fat in your diet. Compare what you learn with the way you normally eat and figure out where you can improve.

Deliberate, measured change requires a different mind-set from the dieter's mentality. In the long run it's much more rewarding, especially as you begin to see positive results and notice improvements. Rather than the ephemeral nature of diets, your new way of eating and preparing foods will become a habit that will last. Soon you'll be able to look back and see how far you've come. You may even catch yourself thinking, "I can't believe I used to eat like that."

Changing the way you eat can be fun if you look at it as a creative challenge. There are many ways to modify your present eating pattern without sacrificing taste or pleasure. A good place to start is by considering what food substitutions you can make without feeling deprived. As you'll see in the following exercise, there are many ways to cut down on fat and make big improvements in your diet.

Exercise: Substitution

Part I
How willing would you be to make the following substitutions or changes? Circle the appropriate mark using the scale below:
1 = I would have no problem making this change.
2 = I'd be willing to try.
3 = I might be willing, but I'm not sure.
4 = I wouldn't like this change very much.
5 = Making this change would definitely make me feel deprived.
N/A = I already do this.

Substitution	Ranking
2% milk for whole milk	1 2 3 4 5 N/A
skim milk for 2% or whole milk	1 2 3 4 5 N/A
reduced-fat margarine for butter	1 2 3 4 5 N/A
nonfat mayonnaise for regular	1 2 3 4 5 N/A
mustard for mayonnaise on sandwiches	1 2 3 4 5 N/A

jelly for butter on toast or bagels	1 2 3 4 5 N/A
vegetable pizza for pepperoni or sausage	1 2 3 4 5 N/A
cooking spray for butter	1 2 3 4 5 N/A
herbs and spices for butter	1 2 3 4 5 N/A
nonfat yogurt for ice cream	1 2 3 4 5 N/A
diet soda for regular	1 2 3 4 5 N/A
nonfat salad dressing for regular	1 2 3 4 5 N/A
pretzels for potato chips	1 2 3 4 5 N/A
nonfat cookies for regular	1 2 3 4 5 N/A
pancakes without butter for buttered pancakes	1 2 3 4 5 N/A
hamburger for cheeseburger	1 2 3 4 5 N/A

Part II

Using your answers from Part I, list the food changes you rated *1* or *2* on the scale (those you could make easily). Also write down any other substitutions not on the list that you would be willing to make on a permanent basis:

_____

_____

_____

Stop! Before you run out and make all the changes you just listed, remember that you want to see lasting progress. The way to do this is to take it slow and easy. Work on making one substitution or change at a time until you're comfortable with it. When you're sure you're not feeling deprived, move on to the next one.

You may choose to substitute low- or nonfat foods for other more fattening choices when you can't tell the difference between nonfat and the real thing. You may end up eliminating certain foods from your diet, but they'll be things you don't mind giving up. By the same token, you may also end up eating your daily honey bun for breakfast if it means that much to you. (Just make sure you account for it by cutting back somewhere else in your day's menu.)

The best way to ensure success is to make sure your new eating habits include foods that satisfy you, even if they aren't what others would consider healthy. The key is to keep your overall diet low in fat and to not exceed your recommended caloric intake, but to still allow yourself enough treats that you never feel deprived. Identify the foods you enjoy, even if they're not normal diet foods, and make them part of your life. You can continue to eat pizza or cake because you'll be listening to your intuition and making choices that feel right.

Whatever you do, don't set rules for yourself that you aren't likely to stick to. Don't force yourself to eat three meals a day if you've never been in the habit of doing so. If you don't normally eat the number of recommended servings of a given food group, don't worry about it. Strive for balance instead.

While you're still in the craving-recovery stage, you may find it helpful to plan in advance what you'll eat each day. Do not, however, confuse this with a diet. The whole point in planning your meals is to eliminate non-hungry snacking that can exacerbate cravings. By planning ahead you'll be ensuring your success by taking control and making sure your day's food supply includes enough to satisfy you mentally and physically. You won't fall into the trap of following a diet designed by someone who doesn't know you and your personal preferences.

In short, make changes you know will work for you. Unless you design your eating plan around your personal schedule and include the foods you prefer, you'll feel deprived and will end up craving the foods you're missing.

To illustrate this point, the following is a typical diet menu. Look it over and think about how it makes you feel:

Breakfast:
1 fruit (½ banana, apple, pear, or 12 grapes)
1 cup skim milk
1 packet instant oatmeal

Lunch:
1 cup low-fat cottage cheese
6 crackers
Salad (lettuce, celery, cucumbers, diet dressing)
Diet drink

Dinner:
4 ounces fish
1 plain baked potato
½ cup vegetables
Tea

Dessert:
½ cup diet Jello

If you really enjoy eating, this menu probably has you shrinking in fear. For a person who struggles with cravings, reading a diet plan like this may have you ready to run screaming to the nearest bag of chocolate chip cookies. The worst part is, you've probably tried to follow a diet just like this at some point in your life, haven't you? How long did you last before your cravings won out?

This menu was designed for the general public. Nutritionally speaking, it's great. It's low calorie, low fat, and well balanced. It includes breakfast, lunch, and dinner and all the major food groups.

And it's boring!

Besides being nearly tasteless, you may have noticed that the previous sample diet didn't include any snacks. The dieter who tries to follow this menu will likely suffer tremendous between-meal cravings, not only because the food is so uninteresting, but because she's not eating enough.

Making long-term changes in your eating habits and giving up dieting does not mean you have to give up snacks. Americans eat three meals a day out of custom and convenience. Unfortunately, your body may not agree with that schedule. You've learned that certain foods give you energy for only a certain number of hours. If you're not eating the right kinds of energy-sustaining foods at frequent enough intervals, you can't be expected to go from one meal to the next without needing, or yes, craving more to eat. Snacking between meals can actually ward off cravings that result from being over hungry.

By listening to your body's hunger signals and asking yourself if you really need to eat, you can make snacking a regular part of your daily food plan. There are, however, a couple of things to keep in mind when it comes to snacking:

- Eating should be a conscious activity. You should be snacking deliberately, rather than mindlessly putting food in your mouth. This is why it's not a good idea to eat while watching TV, driving, or reading. It's too easy to lose track of how much you're eating and end up consuming far more calories than you intended. If you're going to allow yourself the pleasure of snacking, stop all other activities and concentrate on what you're eating. Savor every wonderful mouthful.

- Plan your snacks so that they're healthy and satisfying. Snacks have earned a bad reputation because of the many non-nutritious snack foods available. A large percentage of junk foods are strictly that— junk, consisting of empty calories that sap your energy rather than raise it.

Don't worry, this doesn't mean you have to carry a bag of raw carrots to the office for your mid-afternoon pick-me- up. There are plenty of healthy, nutritional foods from which to choose: low-fat muffins, bagels, nonfat yogurt, pretzels. These days even most vending machines are stocked with good choices.

There's no need to give up the foods that bring you pleasure. You're entitled to eat the foods you like, regardless of how much you weigh or how you look, especially if you remain aware of what your body and your intuition are telling you. The secret is to learn moderation and balance.

Eating a healthy diet is much easier today than it used to be. There's an incredible variety of low- and nonfat foods available (but remember that nonfat doesn't mean non-calorie). Nutritional labels are now on every package, helping you determine if the foods you're buying exceed the 20- 30 percent fat content recommended for a healthy diet.

Grocery stores are full of beautiful fruits and vegetables from all over the world. Bookstores are well stocked with cookbooks that show you how to create lighter versions of your favorite meals. Fancy cafés and even fast food restaurants now offer light meals. Of course, the potato chip and junk food aisles in the local market are overflowing, and fast food restaurants will always rely on burgers, fries, and pizza. But the choice is yours.

You can choose to continue to go on and off diets that don't last, or you can make permanent changes in your eating habits that include your favorite foods. The bottom line is: learn to eat healthy snacks and meals that satisfy you and you'll never have to diet. By making conscious choices about what you eat from one minute to the next, you are practicing total awareness. You're becoming a conscious eater by taking the time to weigh the pros and cons of each food choice.

If you're excited about never having to diet again but are nervous with what may seem like a radical concept, take a deep breath and remember that you can rely on your intuition to make this work. If you find your clothes are getting a little tight, rather than falling back into the diet trap, recognize this as a sign that it's time to slow down and shift gears. Your body is signaling you to take another look at your eating habits. Ask yourself what you've been doing lately that has deviated from your long term healthy eating plan. Make a small change, then find other ways to cut down on fat and increase your activity.

When you're positive you don't feel deprived and you're not struggling, then you can safely try something new. It may take a little longer than you'd like, but every little step you take advances you toward your goal of long-term weight control and the elimination of your cravings.

If you need an extra serving of motivation, try the following affirmations:

I am free of dieting forever.

I am treating myself lovingly by making permanent changes in my lifestyle.

I eat foods that are healthy yet satisfying.

That was the old me—I don't eat like that anymore!

I enjoy my new eating habits.

This is a way of eating I can live with.

I love the new me!

Long-Term Strategy Three: Get active!

In the list of craving quick fixes, you learned how exercise can be an immediate solution to get you through the urge to eat when a craving is at its strongest. Committing yourself to a lifelong exercise program can have even more profound effects on your ability to combat cravings for the long term.

Yes, the preface of this book promised that you wouldn't learn any new exercise routines here, and you won't. But because physical activity can play such a beneficial role in overcoming food cravings, the subject of exercise can't be ignored completely. Becoming more active can be one of the most positive things you can do to treat yourself lovingly as you recover from your obsession with food.

For every negative effect of overeating, exercising produces a positive reaction that can enhance your life in a variety of ways. Some of the great physiological reasons you may want to commit yourself to increasing your activity include:

- lowering your blood pressure
- lowering your cholesterol
- strengthening your muscles, allowing you to handle daily tasks more easily
- increasing your metabolism, helping lower your set point
- helping you recover faster from illnesses
- energizing you

Besides the undeniable benefits to your body, there are the intangible, yet even more valuable advantages exercise offers the food-craver. Instead of stuffing down your emotions with food and suffering from the resultant feelings of guilt and depression, making exercise a regular part of your life:

- helps you handle stress better
- keeps you focused on a healthy lifestyle and healthy food choices
- increases your self-esteem and self-confidence

Do you need any more reasons to get moving?

Many adults rarely get any kind of regular exercise. They have a mental block against it. If this is your problem, the thing to remember is that when it comes to exercise, attitude is everything.

Do you avoid exercise? Have you convinced yourself you hate to work out? Do you think exercise is something only other, more physically fit people do?

If so, your attitude could stem from a life of inactivity. It could even be linked to some very specific events in your childhood.

Maybe you really were the last to be picked for basketball. Maybe you always swung wildly in softball, sure you were going to hit a homer, only to miss the ball completely and be laughed at by the rest of the team. No wonder you have an aversion to exercise. Or perhaps the only time you ever ran was during the yearly physical fitness test in school and it left you gasping for breath and stumbling across the finish line, dead last. Who could blame you for not liking to work out? An untrained body can't run full speed without going into oxygen-deprived agony.

Maybe you don't like to exercise because you're afraid of being ridiculed, of being laughed at, or maybe of looking silly or foolish. Who isn't? The point is, exercise isn't bad, but you may have built up a lot of negative associations with it. People don't like to do things they can't do well, and nobody wants to be made fun of. No one likes pain either, and exercise can definitely bring on discomfort if you do too much, too hard, too soon.

But think back to those times as a kid when exercise was fun. Did you ever roll around in the grass or make snow angels in the yard? Did you ever run around in circles, staring at the clouds until you fell down dizzy and laughing? Did you like to skip? Did you do somersaults in the living room? Did you ride your bike at full speed like a maniac? Did you have a scooter or a wagon? Did you ever move to the beat of a really great song—even if no one was around? Admit it—exercise *can* be fun!

Maybe you haven't allowed yourself to feel how enjoyable exercise can be. It's time to cast off the negative images of exercise that may be holding you back. Just like your other limiting beliefs, the ones you have about exercise may not serve you anymore and are only getting in the way of your health and peace of mind.

Okay, it's true. Play is play and exercise is, well, work—not only to accomplish the physical part, but to keep your motivation up. It may be slow going until you get to the point where you actually enjoy or even look forward to your workout.

While exercise has its moments of drudgery and difficulty, it also has moments of exhilaration. It takes perseverance and commitment, but the payoffs are tremendous: satisfaction, increased energy, better health, less stress, weight loss, a leaner body, and best of all, fewer cravings.

So how do you get past the drudgery? There will always be days that are harder than others, but the key is to find activities you enjoy. Movement feels good. Watch children—they never stop. As any parent knows, kids are perpetual motion machines, always running, skipping, jumping rope, dancing—all great fat-burning, energy-lifting exercises. Choose exercises that let the little kid in you come out.

Enlist a friend to work out with you. Having an exercise partner tends to bring out the competitive nature in people, and you may discover you perform better when working out with a friend than you would if you were by yourself. Companionship alone is enough to make exercising with a partner more enjoyable, but knowing someone else is going to the trouble to get in a workout for the day, you'll be more motivated to put forth the same effort.

If you love music, find or make a tape with a beat that really gets you going. Not only does music help you keep a rhythm or set a pace, it takes your mind off the effort you're exerting! Try the same workout with and without music and see what effect the music has on you.

Nothing will further your efforts and deepen your commitment to exercise like doing things with your body that you never thought possible. Even a little bit of exercise will show you improvements. Set short- and long-term fitness or exercise goals for yourself. Choose something you've never done before, anything from walking around the block to running a ten-kilometer race. Then work toward achieving that goal. Take your focus off food and cravings and put it on something positive.

The day you realize your first fitness goal, no matter how small, you'll be ridding yourself of outdated perceptions of your untrained, unfit self, and deepening your commitment to a lifetime of fitness.

It's incredibly motivating to set a goal and be able to pat yourself on the back after every workout, knowing you're working toward it. Each target you reach becomes one more success to notch in your belt and brag to your friends and family about. Your self-esteem will skyrocket as you create a new image in your mind of the physically fit you.

As you begin to discover the benefits of exercising, you may want to make your workout your number one priority. Let nothing stop you from treating yourself lovingly and taking care of your body before all else.

Here are more ways of making exercise more enjoyable, rather than just tolerable:

1. Don't overdo it. Nothing will set you back or discourage you faster than taking on more than your body can handle. Yes, you may be filled with enthusiasm once you start to feel better about yourself, but parcel that enthusiasm out in little bundles. Save it for the times when you need it most—when your motivation is in need of a boost.

Never exercise to the point where you're completely out of breath. Not only does it cause your body to burn sugar instead of fat, but it's painful and gives exercise a bad name.

Fitness experts recommend that if your goal is to burn fat, you should exercise for a minimum of twelve minutes. You should work at a level where you're breathing heavily, but can still string together three or four words at a time. If you can carry on a normal conversation, you're not exercising hard enough to burn fat, and if you're gasping for breath, you're only burning sugar.

2. If you're uncomfortable about being seen, work out where you won't be

Yes, there may come a time when you want to show the world that you are an exerciser, but if you're not there yet, there are plenty of exercises that can be done in the privacy of your own home. If working out in front of a bunch of women in leotards at a club makes you feel bad, find something else. There are no strict rules about where you have to work out, or with whom. Choose what feels right for you. Wear clothes that are comfortable and make you feel good. There are no rules that say you have to wear tights or skimpy shorts to work out.

3. Find a phrase or thought that motivates you and repeat it during difficult parts of a workout.

Hear your thoughts as you're exercising. Do you constantly tell yourself how miserable you are? Are you concentrating on your discomfort? Your body will act on whatever you tell it. If you convince yourself you can't take another step, suddenly your shoes will feel as if they're filled with lead and you'll come to a dead halt. Instead, make some affirmations for exercise. As you work out, tell yourself such motivating things as:

I know where I've been and I know where I'm going (Your old self versus the leaner, healthier you)

I'm training my body to burn more fat.

I'm treating myself right!

Every step I take is one step closer to my goal.

I'm getting more in shape by the minute!

I am athletic and fit!

I am a runner!

I am a weight lifter, toning and shaping my muscles by the day.

I love working out! (Remember, affirmations work even if they aren't true.)

Have you tried an exercise program in the past but just couldn't stick with it? You can always find a reason not to work out. What's your "exerscuse"?

How often have you told yourself:

Exercise is boring.

I don't have enough time to exercise.

It's raining and I can't work out in the rain.

It's too cold.

I'm too tired.

You may have heard and even used these excuses at least a hundred times. It's easy to make up reasons why you can't get out of your rut and move your body. It takes a lot of effort to put other, less taxing activities aside, change your clothes, and work up a sweat for twenty to thirty minutes, only to have to shower and change back into your clothes. Just like deciding whether to eat a high-fat or nonfat food, whether to give in to a craving or work the four steps of the HALT process, you always have a choice.

Keep your motivation level high and make exercise an easy choice by finding alternate ways of looking at it. Exercise is boring only if you let it be, so jazz it up with music, watch TV while you work out, or buy an energizing workout video.

Vary your workouts. Exercise is much more than just running or aerobics. Why not try cross-country skiing (indoors on a machine or outdoors when it snows), speed-walking, hiking, riding a bike (indoors or out), stair-climbing, jumping rope, rowing, swimming, trampolining, bench-stepping, sliding, skating, playing tennis, roller-blading . . . the list goes on and on.

Choose activities you enjoy. Do the same thing every day if you find it really holds your interest, or do something different every day. Exercise doesn't have to be drudgery.

You don't have time? You could probably make time for something else if you thought it was more enjoyable. When you make your workout your number one priority, it's *other* things you have to find time for.

Find time for exercise by getting up a little earlier in the morning. Exercise while dinner is cooking. Stop going out to lunch or eating at your desk and work out at lunchtime. Exercise in front of the TV in the evening. Twenty to thirty minutes a day, three times a week should be your minimum goal to start reaping the benefits of exercise. Remember—every minute you're exercising is one more minute you're not heading for the refrigerator! And best of all, after treating yourself so lovingly by working out, you'll be much less likely to want to overeat.

It's raining outside? Run anyway! Have fun watching people's faces as you splash through the water. You probably used to deliberately step in puddles as a kid. Get a perverse sense of pleasure out of being one of those crazy people who's out there in any kind of weather (because they care enough to take care of themselves). Okay, so you don't want to get your hair wet? Work out inside. There are plenty of indoor activities. Too cold? Ever go sledding as a kid? Do you ski? It's never too cold for that, is it? Dress for the weather and you'll be fine. It's amazing how technologically advanced cold-weather workout clothes have become. Just like the first shock of jumping into a cold swimming pool, your body adjusts quickly to the environment, especially as you warm up through exercise. Take the plunge and get moving!

Too tired? Exercise is exactly what you need to get your blood flowing again. Sometimes it can take a super-human effort to drag your tired body off the couch after a stressful day at work, but the invigoration you'll feel after twenty to thirty minutes of fat-burning exercise can erase a whole day of aggravation. You may feel tired when you finish your workout, but it's a different kind of tired from the kind you get from stress or inactivity.

You'll be clear-headed and alert, and you'll feel terrific because you took care of your number one priority—you.

If you move long enough and hard enough in your workouts, you may experience that extra special benefit of exercise known as the "runner's high." You don't have to run a marathon to experience the rush of good feelings that comes from a good workout. In response to extended physical effort, the brain releases chemicals called *endorphins*. These self-manufactured painkillers can make you feel like Rocky, and are one of the reasons people who get hooked on exercise keep coming back for more.

Although some people take exercise to an extreme, you can find an exercise program that doesn't exhaust you, yet leaves you feeling great. Replacing your cravings with this kind of addiction is a very wise choice.

It may take months, or even years, until working out becomes more a pleasure than a chore. If you stick with it, however, you'll notice a gradual change in your attitude toward exercise. It will become a part of your life, to the point where it's more than just a way to lose weight. Exercise will enrich your body and your soul so that if you go more than a couple of days without working out, you'll feel sluggish and irritable.

When faced with the daily decision of whether to exercise or not, ask yourself if you want to remain the way you are, or if you want to treat yourself lovingly. The benefits of exercise extend far beyond the physical, positively affecting every other aspect of your life.

If you're ready to make some permanent, positive lifestyle changes, take the advice of the experts who make Nike shoes— JUST DO IT!

Long-Term Strategy four: Relax your standards.

Do you find you constantly grade yourself on how you do things? Do you feel pressured to do everything flawlessly? Perhaps you've been accused of being a perfectionist. If so, your drive to do everything "the right way" may be sabotaging your efforts to stop obsessing about food.

Even if you have no problem leaving a few dirty clothes lying around on the floor or don't feel every hair on your head has to be in place, don't skip this section. Many cravers can have relaxed standards in other aspects of their lives, yet be perfectionists when it comes to the way they eat.

Cravers often suffer from a type of all-or-nothing thinking about food. They feel as if they've failed if they eat something they consider bad. Eating is either black or white, with no gray area in between. One minor digression can lead to an entire day of unhealthy eating. Three grapes can constitute a binge to a perfectionistic eater. If you are an all-or-nothing eater, the first thing you need to do is hear the limiting beliefs that keep you subscribing to this attitude. The second thing you can do is treat yourself lovingly and relax your standards. Determine what requirements you place on yourself that create the feeling of failure. You may have set goals about your eating habits that are unrealistic.

If you believe you have to eat healthy, low-fat foods twenty-four hours a day, seven days a week, then your expectations are achievable but unreasonable. By believing you have to eat perfectly 100 percent of the time, you'll feel like a failure anytime you eat a non-healthy treat (and there are plenty of them our there). Eating junk food on occasion or allowing yourself to indulge in desserts is perfectly acceptable and normal behavior.

Whether you eat healthy foods 100 percent, 80 percent, 60 percent, 50 percent, or 20 percent of the time, you are still a loveable, worthy human being. Treat yourself lovingly and allow yourself not to be perfect.

Until now you probably haven't been eating right all the time anyway, have you? What's the longest rime you ever went without eating something you considered bad? What good did it do you? Did you end up feeling deprived? Did you compensate for the deprivation by overeating? Food is not good or bad. It's just food.

Perfectionistic eating serves no beneficial purpose. By expecting too much of yourself, you place undue pressure that can only add to your desire to eat. From now on, every time you become aware that you're berating yourself for not being a perfect eater or for not resisting your cravings 100 percent of the time, ask yourself, "What difference does it make in the grand scheme of things?" Adjust your eating habits to allow for enjoyment, and let go of the need to be perfect.

Practice acceptance and forgiveness. You're not perfect. You're human. Accept your imperfections. It's OK to expect more of yourself than you would expect of someone else, but be reasonable. All you can ask of yourself is to do your best.

Part V
Putting It All Together

16

Reviewing the Process

As you recall, people who are unaware of the cause of their cravings tend to eat unconsciously. Their actions trap them in the craving cycle, enslaving them in the typical chain of events you're now familiar with. Using the HALT strategies as your ammunition, you're now able to end this self-defeating cycle by bringing subconscious thoughts, feelings, and actions to the surface.

By putting everything you've learned into practice, you're able to get off the treadmill by responding to cravings from a position of power:

- You become aware of a craving and call an immediate HALT.
- You recognize your self-defeating thoughts and turn them around.
- You pay attention to the feelings your thoughts are triggering, calling on your counselor to help you feel them, if necessary.
- You accept all your emotions, good and bad, recognizing that they may be showing you an area in your life that needs to be changed. Having done so, you let them wash through you.
- You recognize you have valid needs that aren't necessarily being met. You accept responsibility for your needs and you take action to change things that leave you feeling unfulfilled. If the craving persists:
- You recognize from your body and your mental signals that you are still struggling.
- You realize the reason you're struggling is because your intuition is trying to tell you something and you're not listening. You relinquish control and turn over your struggle to your inner guide.

- You ask yourself what would feel good at that moment and stay tuned for an answer.
- If you're feeling particularly stressed or out of contact with your inner guide, you take a few minutes for yourself and meditate.
- You find a positive alternative to eating and give yourself a big pat on the back for taking care of yourself.
- You do your best to treat yourself with kindness and love throughout the day.

While your new method of dealing with cravings appears time-consuming, with practice it will actually take less time than you used to spend fighting your cravings. The result of a little extra effort now is a permanent end to the cycle that in the past only brought you pain.

The biggest change from your former ways is the sense of awareness and power you have when you use the HALT process. Your old pattern was a series of subconscious thoughts that left you feeling out of control. The New You knows that to conquer your cravings you have to be much more conscious of everything that is going on in your mind and body. You need to work with, instead of against, yourself.

Being fully aware means constantly asking yourself questions about your thoughts, your feelings, your needs, your physical sensations, and what's going on around you. It means making a dedicated effort to help yourself get better, rather than waiting for improvements to happen by themselves.

Until personal awareness becomes second nature, it may help to carry around a HALT checklist. Write out each of the four steps and make up a corresponding set of questions for each of them. The following list is only a sampling of things you can include on your checklist to increase your awareness when faced with a craving:

Hear your thoughts:

- What am I thinking right now?
- What voices are talking to me?
- What am I telling myself?
- Are my inner messages actually true?

- What am I thinking about my body?
- What's really making me want to eat?

Allow yourself to feel:

- Am I really hungry?
- What emotions am I feeling?
- Is there something I need?
- Do I crave food or just attention?
- How will I feel later if I eat now?
- What emotions do I need to accept and act on?
- How can I take charge of my life?

Listen to your intuition:

- Is my body telling me I'm struggling? Why?
- Am I anxious? (Am I struggling mentally?)
- Are my inner voices friendly or destructive?
- Am I out of touch with my intuition?
- Do I need to meditate or take some time for myself?
- Am I listening to my inner messages?
- Am I giving myself permission to eat or am I still restricting myself?
- What would feel better right now rather than eating?

Treat yourself lovingly:

- How am I treating myself?
- Am I talking to myself like a friend?
- Am I taking time to do enjoyable things and be good to myself?
- Am I balancing work with play?
- Am I taking care of myself physically?
- Am I expecting the best and working to achieve it?

Depending on your particular needs and circumstances, not every one of the steps in the HALT process will be as meaningful as another to you in a given situation. Therefore, it's important to focus on those that strike the deepest chord inside. Select the craving-fighters you feel will work best for you and tailor your checklist to your particular needs. Ask yourself which area needs the most work and focus your awareness there. After you've used your list a few times, asking yourself these prepared questions and working through the HALT process will become second nature.

Now that you know the cause of your cravings, you'll find you're automatically examining your thought processes and are working to understand why you behave the way you do. By applying the four steps continuously, you'll face your food fears. As you face your fears, they'll disappear, and you'll be able to deal with your eating habits and any underlying issues in a more healthy manner than by overeating.

Before you know it, you'll begin to react to food in ways which before were completely unimaginable. Because of your increased awareness and the effort you're expending, you'll discover your old reactions to food are changing. You may walk by a candy machine and realize you no longer tense up in fear of going on a binge. Instead, you may catch yourself thinking, "I don't buy that stuff anymore." Moments like these will show you all your efforts are paying off.

17
Paperwork

Nothing can provide you better focus as you work toward your recovery from food obsession than to put pen to paper. The simple act of writing down your thoughts and feelings brings them to the forefront and keeps you moving in the right direction. An excellent way to improve your awareness and get more in touch with yourself is to keep a craving journal.

Use a journal to document your successes and your failures. When you find yourself thinking new, empowering phrases or acting in ways that are a complete change from the old you, your journal will provide a written record of your progress. By writing down your achievements, you'll be able to celebrate and congratulate yourself on what's working. Conversely, if you continue to be interrupted by negative, incorrect thoughts that work against you, putting them in a journal and reviewing them from time to time will point out what you still need to work on.

Journaling is easy. You simply write whatever you want, whenever you want. Write often. Try to make an entry in your journal at least once a day during your craving recovery. Do not, however, use it as another way to beat yourself up if you don't get around to writing on a regular basis. Journaling should be a positive and enjoyable experience.

Start each new entry with the day, month, and year. This will help you gauge how quickly you're improving in your relationship with food. Don't worry if your penmanship isn't the best. Don't worry about grammar, punctuation, or writing in complete sentences either; your tenth grade English teacher isn't going to grade it. In fact, that's the great thing about a journal: nobody is going to read it unless you want them to. You can write whatever you want, however you want. It's your private diary with your private thoughts. You are writing for you.

You can journal at any time. Write while you're eating breakfast. Take your journal to work with you and add to it throughout the day. Take a few peaceful minutes for yourself in the evening and spend them writing. Reread your journal before going to bed.

The very best time to write is when you're in the grip of a craving. Since the purpose of keeping a journal is to increase your self-awareness, there's no better way to hear your thoughts and allow yourself to feel than to grab a pencil and work through the HALT process on paper. Not only will your craving journal keep you more focused on your recovery, but it will make the four steps that much more familiar to you.

Jot down your thoughts as you hear them. Write the things you're telling yourself word for word, even if you know they're counterproductive. Write down what you were doing before the craving came on and explore why it triggered what you're feeling at that moment. Ask yourself in writing if you're really hungry. Write down everything you're feeling as you experience the craving.

Have a conscious mental dialogue on paper. Write down which voices are dominating and how you deal with them. Keep working through the craving and ask yourself how you'll feel later if you give in to your present desires. If you're upset with yourself for having the craving, get angry in writing. Notice what kinds of things you're telling yourself. Let your written words show you where the craving you're suffering originated and what's keeping it going. Write down how your body feels. Where's your tension?

Making entries when you're actually having a craving may be the most effective use of a journal, but it's not always possible or convenient to take notes right when the urge to eat hits. If you're in the middle of something that doesn't allow you to stop and write, make a mental note to record your thoughts at a more appropriate time. Just knowing you're going to be writing about your craving later will increase your awareness and help you turn your thoughts around right then and there. Then, when you do have a few minutes, write about what led to your craving and how you handled it. Did you move on to something more productive or did you give in to it and eat? If so, why? Record everything.

A journal doesn't have to be limited to exploring your cravings. As you've learned, there are many issues and themes that cause a person to overeat. Use your journal to examine any concerns in your life that may be contributing to your preoccupation with food.

If you don't know what else to write about, the following ideas, along with some sample entries, may give you food for thought:

- Explore your emotions in depth. This is especially helpful for people who have trouble expressing anger. Give particular attention to any suppressed feelings you're uncomfortable with or have difficulty expressing to others. Here's a journal entry as an example: *What am I feeling? There's a sense of hopelessness and fear. It's very scary. Calf muscles are tight. Arms and shoulders are tense. Teeth are clenched. Stomach is in knots. Breathing shallow. Why? What am I thinking about? I hate this feeling. I don't want to be like this. Could it be I'm afraid all these new things aren't going to work? What's the worst that could happen? I could go back to the way I was. I could completely give up all belief and trust in my inner power and go back to feeling miserable, heavy, and dull. I could have constant cravings forever. I am not going to let that happen! I will learn to trust myself. I will use my affirmations. I will be completely comfortable with myself. I will no longer worry. Wow. Just thought of something. . . maybe I'm afraid of changing my old habits! I'm not comfortable with them, but I'm used to them. Time to let go!*

- Write about your slipups—those times when you gave in and ate when you really didn't want to. Be very careful, however, not to let these entries trigger a chain of negative emotions. Use them as the learning tools they are. Find out what led you to overeat, then determine how you can do better next time.
  Really wanted to eat those onion rolls when I got back from lunch. Wasn't even hungry, but I ate all three. Didn't listen to my body. Realize now that I wasn't tuned in to my Self. Need to listen. Need to ask myself questions.

- Write down any interaction or conversations you have with your inner guide, even if they aren't related to your cravings. Record the questions you ask and the answers you receive.

Must stop fighting my intuition and learn to trust it. Last night before I ate too much. I was concentrating completely on the craving. When I asked myself if it would feel okay to go ahead and eat, I felt a definite "no." Shut out the voice. Didn't want to hear it. Went back to my old programming. Didn't bother to ask what would feel good right now and follow through on it.

- Write to the different voices in you, such as the craver, the parent, the little kid who's feeling deprived.

  I know I haven't been paying much attention to you lately. All I do is work. Been having lots of cravings lately. Maybe you've been trying to let me know you need to have some fun. Don't worry. Things are going to change around here.

- Your journal is a place to feel safe to express yourself. Have a written dialogue with people who are causing you stress. Vent on paper:

  John, I can't stand it when you come home and expect me to do all the cooking and cleaning by myself. We both work all day. Maybe we need to talk more about this.

- Write about things that happened during the day that brought out strong emotions. This can be something positive or negative. How did it affect you? How did you deal with it?

  John had another one of his temper tantrums today and I realized 1 was letting his anger affect me. It was his problem, but I got upset. I was taking on his negative emotions, even though I'd been in a good mood up until then. For the first time I let them flow through me. Didn't block them. Was able to separate his feelings from mine. It worked!

- Write about any resentments you're keeping bottled up inside. Explore how you could let go of them.

  Can't stand when Mary uses that tone of voice with me. Why can't I just tell her? There must be a way to deal with this that won't alienate her. This may make a good question to ask next time I meditate.

140

- Write down the details about any problems or conflicts you're having in any area of your life, not just those related to food. The simple act of writing them down makes your subconscious mind more open to solutions.

  Why can't I find the time to do everything I want to do in a day? Everything keeps piling up. There's got to be a better way to ease some of this pressure than eating.

- Delve into any self-esteem issues you're dealing with. Try to find the fallacies in your thoughts.

  Interesting. . . one of my main goals was to fit comfortably in the size eight pants I bought for my visit to Kathy's house. Well, I did it! (Good for me!) But the funny thing is, neither Kathy nor her mother (nor anybody!) commented on how I looked. There I was, all obsessed about the weight I lost, and it didn't make the slightest difference to anyone! They were interested in me for me! Wow!

Your journal shouldn't be completely negative. Keep your writing balanced by including such issues as:

- Things that make you feel good about yourself.

  Had two lousy days. Was ready to give up everything, then it hit me! I've felt bad ever since I stepped on the scales two days ago. Wasn't trusting myself and thought I needed the scales to show me how I was doing. I let the numbers influence me! Now I realize all that really matters is how I feel about myself. Those are just numbers. Clothes are fitting better than before. The second I decided to get rid of my scales for good I felt wonderful! I don't ever need them again. Need to thank my inner guide for not abandoning me and helping me to see this.

- Praise for yourself and encouragement in your recovery.

  This stuff is really working! As my body learns I'll feed it what it wants, when it wants, I'm able to relax. Seems like more and more I only want the foods that are good for me. Guess I'm doing better than I thought I would.

- Signs of The New You.

  Realized that yesterday there were Girl Scout cookies in the kitchen cupboard and I had no desire to eat them. I even forgot they were there.

Now that's a first! Didn't even realize at the time how natural that felt. This is becoming part of me already. Gotta keep working at it!

- Things you're looking forward to.
  We're all going out to dinner tonight to celebrate Joe's promotion. Can't wait to actually enjoy a meal rather than worrying about what I'm going to eat or what everybody else is having. I give myself permission to eat anything, as long as my intuition tells me it's okay. Can't believe how good it feels to know I won't feel tortured to eat dessert.

You may have noticed that several of these journal entries focused on how well the writer was doing in her recovery from cravings. The importance of writing about your successes can't be stressed enough. Record every victory you achieve in your battle with cravings, no matter how big or small. Give yourself high praise for getting through a situation in which you would normally have overeaten. Recognize this as yet another triumph and reread these particular pages in your journal to reinforce your efforts whenever you need encouragement:

Mike brought in a dozen doughnuts today. They might as well have been a pile of rocks sitting there. They held no power over me. Never would have reacted like that before. Felt so strong! It works! Ate a cookie when I got home from work. Afterward I wanted to eat more and more and more. Felt the same old conflict—very intense. The craving voice was so strong it almost overpowered my intuition. Stopped and recognized the fear of totally losing control. Listened for my intuition, turned the fear over to her, and the craving vanished immediately! I feel great!

As you can see, a chronicle of your recovery gives you a written record to look at as time passes so you can see just how far you've come. You'll be able to read over your pages and observe the daily progress you make. Comparing the earlier pages to your most recent, you'll notice improvements in your thoughts and in your habitual reactions to food. Your writings will be proof positive that you're making the HALT process work. If you're committed to your journal and make regular entries, you'll experience an interesting phenomenon. After journaling for a few weeks, you'll begin to notice recurring themes when you write about your cravings. The same thoughts will keep repeating themselves. You'll realize you're beginning to sound like a broken record. It won't take long before you start to get tired of writing these phrases over and over.

For a recovering food-craver, this can be a turning point. Once you recognize that your craving thoughts all sound alike, they'll begin to lose their power. You'll see just how poorly they serve you and you'll understand how you've been falsely programming your mind. This is the beauty of being a conscious eater and is what makes journaling worth all the time and effort you put into it.

Start writing as soon as you can. You can use a plain notebook, but why not treat yourself to a journal with an attractive or interesting cover? (Just like a gift you'd give your best friend.) You can find decorative blank books in almost any bookstore or card shop.

Unless you're afraid someone is going to read it, keep your journal somewhere you'll be sure to see it and use it often, such as on the night stand next to your bed. Once you begin to discover the benefits of journaling, you may even end up carrying your book with you in a purse or briefcase.

Keeping a journal is part of your commitment to you. It is one of the most valuable tools you will use in your recovery. Another type of book you can create for yourself is a personal collection of power thoughts.

Find a blank notepad that's small enough to carry anywhere. While you can easily include your power thoughts in a separate section of your journal, it may serve you better to keep these highly motivational phrases in their own special book. In it you will write all the short yet powerful thoughts and ideas relating to your recovery from food obsession that really hit home. These can be full-sentence affirmations, or they can include shorter bursts of enthusiastic, motivational words. Any time you think of an idea or read a craving-fighting suggestion that strikes a special chord in you, add it to your book.

Here are just a few examples of power phrases that you may want to include in your book:

HALT!
I've got the power!
I don't do that anymore!
That was the old me!
I control my thoughts!

Food has no power!
Trust!

As you find your motivators, give each its own page in your book. Write these super sentences in big, bold letters. Highlight them in different colors, underline them, but most of all, use them! Carry the book with you in your purse or pocket and pull it out any time you need an extra dose of inspiration.

A lot of the things you're doing now to conquer your cravings may be a totally new way of behaving or thinking. Your personal power phrases are the heavy ammunition you can pull out when you need to feel good instantly. If you find yourself in the middle of a craving and need a little help getting through it, it's great to know where to turn to stay on target.

18

Success and Setbacks

All successful people have one thing in common: they don't quit. They persevere, even when they encounter setbacks. They're committed to reaching their goals. Successful people have learned to conquer the temptation to give up. Winners also share another characteristic. They feel passionate about what they're going after. Their desire to achieve success is intense.

How strongly do you want to be rid of your cravings? How much does the thought of being free motivate you? Use that fiery emotion and determination to your benefit. Harness it and let it propel you to put your new strategies to use. Substitute all the energy you used to put into fighting your cravings for the energy needed to do your inner work.

If you can see your success, you can achieve it. Be your own cheerleader. Make recovery your number one priority. Get excited! Have faith in yourself. Are you willing to put forth every bit of effort you have for the peace of mind that awaits you? Are you willing to put up with setbacks and disappointments in exchange for freedom from your chronic preoccupation with food? Do you have the determination and motivation to succeed?

There's no sugarcoating it: the end to your battle with cravings is an uphill climb. The road, however, does not go straight up. It's more like a chain of mountains with high points, low points, and some plateaus. Success requires perseverance and tenacity and an acceptance that there will be rough spots.

If you want to be successful in conquering your cravings, you must *expect* setbacks. Be prepared for them. Have the right tools readily accessible when you encounter them. Learn to accept them and deal with them, but even more important, learn from them.

You may think you've almost reached your mountaintop, when you'll suddenly find yourself slipping backward. Just when you think you can deal with any food situation, you may get a massive craving and give in to it, resorting to your old ways. A quitter would consider this a major failure and would wipe out all the good efforts she'd made in getting to that point. She would probably consider herself a failure as well and would allow all her old self-defeating thoughts and self-talk to flow right back in.

Winners use setbacks as learning experiences. Setbacks can show you what you still need to work on. They produce patience and serve as reality checks. If you give in to a craving and overeat when you don't really want to, do what winners do. Take time to figure out what happened, then adjust your actions to keep from doing the same thing again later.

You've done the preparation and you have all the right tools at your disposal. You've rooted out your negative thinking and have a list of motivating affirmations. You are actively visualizing your success. You know how to stop and meditate when the going gets stressful. You have a journal to give you reinforcements, and you'll be accompanied by your own personal guide every step of the way.

When you experience the inevitable setbacks, be sure to treat yourself lovingly. Just as you would never scold a child for falling down while learning to walk, give yourself encouragement instead of criticism if you stumble.

To reach your goal, you'll have to exercise not just your body, but your mind. Old habits die hard, so train yourself to apply your new strategies. Have daily mental workouts. Think through how you will deal with any problems you may encounter. The need to work so hard will trail off as all your new thoughts and actions become second nature.

If you resolve not to quit and to learn from your mistakes, success *will* be yours. Feel it. See it. Know it.

It's often been said that "winners never quit and quitters never win." The people who give up in their battle against cravings do so because it's harder than they thought it would be. When they have setbacks and things aren't going as well as they thought they would, they surrender. The key is to remain focused and never lose sight of your goal. Always give your personal best.

You can't ask more of yourself than that.

19

Your Plan of Attack

Knowing what makes a person successful isn't enough. Success doesn't happen by itself. To win your battle with cravings, you must *plan* to succeed. All the tips and strategies in this book are useless unless you make a commitment to use them and come up with a way to incorporate them into your daily life.

As you just learned, successful people are goal oriented. They know what they want and every action they take is directed at going for it. If they get off course, they figure out where they went wrong, then readjust and try again.

To conquer your cravings, you will achieve your objective much sooner and with much more ease if you set specific, craving-related goals for yourself. Even though you know in your heart and your mind what you want to achieve, you will also have much greater success if you put those visions on paper.

Because your intent is to focus all your efforts on the desired outcome, your goal statements must be written down to have the greatest impact. Your journal is a perfect place for your craving related goals.

When writing your goals, there are a few guidelines you should follow to ensure they serve their intended purpose. First, they should be realistic. After reading this book and trying a few of the techniques, you should be forming a new idea of what you're truly capable of achieving. You may have small doubts and fears about your ability to do something you've never done before, but you should also know what is and isn't possible. Don't choose a goal that is asking too much of yourself too soon.

And that leads directly to the second guideline: make your goals time specific. Give yourself a deadline that leaves you enough time to achieve your goal, but is not so far away that you lose motivation. Dreams have a way of slipping away. If you fail to attach a date by which you will achieve your goal, it becomes too easy to ignore. Even if the date you set for yourself is a year away, that date will get here much sooner than "some day."

Finally, make sure your goal statements excite you. You'll never make the effort required to achieve them if you subconsciously find your goals boring. They should really motivate you. Find objectives that fire you up and which you truly feel committed to achieving.

As with everything else you plan for in life, you should have both long-term and short-term craving-related goals. The long-term ones will represent the ultimate "you" you're working to achieve. The smaller goals will be the stepping stones that will get you there. Each time you achieve one of your smaller goals, you'll be even more motivated to continue working for the big payoff.

You may never set a goal to run a marathon, but what's your marathon when it comes to cravings? What personal races are you willing to run to get to your finish line? It's time to come up with your own goals to achieve your personal victory over cravings. To help you, turn back to the first page of the introduction. Read again about the life you were asked to imagine.

It's the kind of life you're hoping for, isn't it?

Did anything on that list represent something you've always dreamed of being able to do? You've now learned the four steps in the HALT process and have had a few successes applying the many strategies that go along with them. Do you see a flicker of light that the kinds of behaviors on the list could be the way you'll be acting in very short order?

That list represents a person who has overcome her past problems and is free of her preoccupation with food. It represents someone who relates to food in a healthy, realistic manner. Any one of these items would make an excellent long-term goal and may be one you want to tailor to yourself. Rewritten in goal-statement form, these phrases would read something like this:

- By Christmas day I will be able to get through a whole evening at home without wondering if there's anything good to eat in the kitchen.
- I will be able to go to Jane's party on April 30 and be more interested in what she and my friends have to say than what's on the buffet table.
- At the start of the school year, I will be the person I've always dreamed of and will be able to take just one bite of any dessert without being afraid of overeating afterward.

Notice how all of these goal statements have built-in time lines. They not only give you a desired outcome on which to focus, but they let you know you'd better get to work if you're going to make it come true.

So how are you going to achieve your long-term goals? You're going to do it by applying the tactics you've learned in this book. If any that you've tried so far have worked better than others, you'll want to concentrate on those and turn them into individual short-term goals. If you've had good success already with your new affirmations, make yourself a promise such as, "I will repeat my list of affirmations every night before going to bed for at least three weeks."

This is something you can easily accomplish. It's also something that unless it's written down and you make a commitment to doing it, can slip through the cracks and be forgotten. Making it into a short-term goal and putting it in writing makes this activity much harder to ignore.

Or how about, "I will meditate at least thirty minutes every day for one month." Okay, this goal has a time line, but is it reasonable? Make sure you design your goals with your lifestyle in mind. If your normal day consists of rushing from one thing to another until you collapse into bed at night, this may not be an achievable goal. You want to succeed at your goals, so if you truly want to make meditation a part of your life, figure out how much time you can reasonably expect to devote to it. Is it something you really want to do every day? Great! But thirty minutes might be a bit ambitious. Once again, give your goals a sanity check.

Your short-term goals can include dedicating yourself to writing in your journal, creating a new exercise plan, or making gradual changes in your eating habits. Take a hard look at your long-term goal and figure out what it's going to take to get you there. Make it as easy as you can by giving yourself milestones along the way by which you can measure your progress.

Your short-term goals make up your plan of action. They will help you maneuver through any minefields that may lie between you and your ultimate goal of peace of mind and freedom from cravings. Review and reaffirm your short-term goals every day to maintain your focus. Constantly see yourself achieving them and your actions will follow.

You can find time to meditate. You can write in a journal. You can remember to call a HALT. This is easy stuff! You can actually *see* yourself being successful at these things. Best of all, these small, easily achievable goals that you set for yourself will lead you straight to your long-term goal and will make it seem less overwhelming.

Exercise: Goal-Setting

Use this space to list your long-term goals. Focus on specific craving-related behaviors you intend to overcome. Be time specific.

_____

_____

_____

_____

Now devise a plan of attack. This is your list of short-term goals, made up of individual strategies and activities you've learned for dealing with your cravings.

_____

_____

_____

_____

Now that you've identified a set of short- and long-term goals that will work for you, you can take your list and go one step further. Combine your long-term goals and expand them into a full vision of how your world will be when all these goals become your reality (and they will).

For the best results, write your vision statement in the present tense. For example, "I am now living my life the way I have always wanted to. I am free of cravings. I . . . (you fill in the rest) . Describe how you will act, as if you're acting that way now. How do you feel in your new life? How do you deal with food? How do you handle negative emotions? How do you feel about yourself?

The following exercise is provided for you to rewrite your goal statements and form your vision of The New You, incorporating all the things you've learned about yourself in this book and all the changes you want to make in your life.

Address the new ways you want to think and act, not just regarding food, but in any areas in which you'd like to improve. After you've filled it in, read it over and make sure it excites you. Remember, even if you don't believe it's possible, it should reflect exactly the "you" you've been dreaming of. Keep in mind that you will act on whatever you tell yourself. In this way, your vision statement becomes your most powerful affirmation. It becomes your very own self-fulfilling prophecy.

Exercise: Vision

In the space below, fill in your personal long-term goals for the future regarding you and your cravings.
My goals are to:

_____

_____

_____

Now describe in detail in the present tense how your world will be when these goal statements are your reality.
I am now living my life the way I've always wanted to. I . . .

_____

_____

_____

_____

Once you're happy with your vision statement, put it where you'll read it often. Read it over and over until it becomes part of you. Visualize yourself becoming the person you've written about.

You may grow tired of reading the same words and put the page away. The wonderful thing is, if you continue to apply the HALT principles, some day you'll stumble across your goal statement and find that you're living the words on the page. Your goals really will have become your reality.

20
The Future

So now you're ready to do battle. You fully expect success because you've now had some previously unimagined personal victories as a result of using the things you've learned. You know what to do and you have a plan of attack. You're committed to applying the HALT strategies. But what if your cravings don't stop right away?

The best advice you can give yourself at this moment, besides getting rid of all the fearful what ifs, is this: be patient with yourself. You didn't develop your habit of thinking negatively, suppressing your feelings, and medicating yourself with food overnight. Your cravings grew out of a lifetime of not treating yourself lovingly. You need to be realistic, as well as forgiving, and expect slipups from time to time.

In addition to being patient, as you apply your new strategies be sure you focus on your successes rather than dwelling on the past. You wouldn't have read this book if you didn't have a problem with food. But that was before you knew how to handle your cravings. You ought to be excited! Today really is the first day of the rest of your life ..your life without cravings.

As you work at your recovery, there's no need to block out your past behaviors and pretend they didn't happen. That was an important part of you. Your cravings and your reactions to them served a purpose by getting you where you are today. But now keep your focus on where you want to go with your plan instead of reminding yourself where you've been. Consider today a fresh starting point from which to move forward.

It's time to forgive yourself for all the times you dealt with food in ways other than you intended. Forgive yourself for having been a craver. Use that part of your life as a learning experience and move on. Who you were in the past and how you acted around food is not who you are now. Now that you're allowing yourself to hear your thoughts and feel your emotions, you're making positive changes and learning from your mistakes. You're no longer working alone, but are getting better with the help of your intuition.

Treat yourself lovingly and reward yourself for each victory in your battle with cravings. Every time you do something that in the past you thought was impossible, recognize it as a major accomplishment and give yourself praise and encouragement. Get rid of old baggage. Update worn-out images of yourself. Think of things you used to do or used to eat that you know weren't good for you and proclaim proudly, "I don't do that anymore!" It makes no difference how you behaved in the past. That was the old you.

If curing your cravings were as easy as reading this book from front to back, the diet industry would be out of business. Unfortunately, the real work is just beginning. It will take a lot of effort and real dedication to apply what you've learned, but you already have the desire to change or you wouldn't have read this far.

If a craving hits, don't panic. Sift through the myriad of options you now have at your disposal and you'll get through it. The next time you get a craving you'll be that much better prepared to deal with it. Before you know it, you'll notice that the time between cravings is increasing while your fear of them is decreasing.

For as long as you've been suffering, your focus has been on food and your preoccupation with it. Now that your focus is shifting to your recovery, your thoughts will be filled with all your new ideas and images. Ever so slowly you'll notice that eating and your recovery from cravings will take up less of your time and attention.

As you become less preoccupied with food, you'll find that your attention is moving from a predominantly inward focus to one where you look beyond yourself. You'll feel more connected with others and the world around you than ever before because you're far less self-concerned. You'll be more able to love others more because you love yourself more.

As a result of being in tune with your intuitive side, your creative juices will flow more freely. You'll find more pleasant ways to enjoy your free time and will search for imaginative outlets for your newfound energy and enthusiasm. You'll discover a passion for life that's been buried beneath the surface, just waiting to be set free.

You'll realize you are creating your own happiness rather than letting others do it for you. Your satisfaction will come from inside, rather than from what others do or say. Whereas in the past you derived most of your happiness from simple, short-lived amusement, you'll find yourself looking for enjoyable pursuits that provide more of a sense of purpose or mission.

If your relationships are troublesome or your job isn't satisfying, you'll no longer turn to food as a way of avoiding your problems. You'll be much more willing to face your troubles head-on and make positive changes, rather than returning to a lifestyle that didn't serve you.

Your recovery from cravings will be a wonderful journey of self-discovery as you uncover a new and powerful you that's been hiding beneath the surface.

Don't doubt it. Just trust yourself, relax, and enjoy the process.

Appendix A
Recognizing Eating Disorders

Some people from time to time demonstrate behaviors that are representative of eating disorders, such as eating in secret or obsessing about weight. While this type of behavior is not desirable, it's not life-threatening and can be treated through the various self-help methods discussed in this book. The following actions, however, are indicative of a more serious problem than a fixation with food.

People who suffer from anorexia:
- turn away from food to cope with their problems
- have trouble concentrating
- have dry or pale skin for no apparent reason (it's not related to illness or weather)
- often get light-headed and may feel close to fainting
- get cold easily
- stop having menstrual periods
- lose a lot of weight over a short period of time (and it's not due to other illness)
- are often constipated
- have brittle nails
- weigh themselves frequently
- binge (yes, that's right—up to half of all anorexics binge)
- exercise to excess (more than two hours at a time on a regular basis, especially as a response to having recently eaten)

- use exercise mostly as a means to control weight rather than to achieve physical fitness
- are afraid of food and try to stay away from it
- choose clothes to hide their weight loss or buy clothes that show off how much they've lost
- panic at the thought of getting fat, but their idea of "fat" may differ from the norm
- eat very little; others often comment that they are not eating enough
- play with their food, making it look like they're eating when they're really not
- refuse to eat, even though they're actually very hungry
- have mealtime rituals, such as always cutting food into tiny, equally sized pieces
- see themselves as overweight when they look in a mirror, even though they may be extremely thin or emaciated
- want to be alone most of the time
- are perfectionists and feel a need to maintain control
- suffer from severe mood swings, usually related to what and how much they eat
- strongly deny their weight loss and other symptoms

People who suffer with bulimia:
- turn to food to cope with their problems
- binge, consuming excessive quantities of food
- purge themselves by vomiting or using laxatives, diuretics (water pills), enemas, or excessive exercise
- may have dental problems
- get light-headed and disoriented
- suffer from flu-like symptoms such as headaches, fatigue, sore throats, and muscle aches
- may frequently have broken blood vessels under their eyes
- have fluctuating weight losses and gains, but often remain within the normal weight range
- are inordinately afraid of getting fat
- eat quickly and often visit the bathroom shortly after eating

- talk a lot about food and weight-related issues
- occasionally fast
- run short on money from spending available cash on large purchases of food
- steal food
- do most of their eating in private
- have big mood swings related to their eating
- have an inordinately strong need for others' approval

If you feel your eating is out of control to the point where you're hurting yourself physically, or you can no longer handle your mental distress on your own, you should consult a professional counselor. Your best bet is to find someone who is experienced and knowledgeable in the treatment of eating disorders. A good place for information on sources of help nearest you is the National Eating Disorders Association: http:// www.nationaleatingdisorders.org. Their helpline is 1-800-931-2237

Appendix B
Additional Affirmations

The following are affirmations, arranged to coincide with each chapter, that will help reinforce everything you've learned in this book. Read through the entire list, highlighting those that excite and energize you the most, and add these to your list.

Remember: your affirmations don't have to be true for you now. If you want them to describe the "you" you desire to become, simply use them. Your actions will follow. Soon they really will be a reflection of who you are.

Cravings and Thoughts
• My cravings are nothing more than thoughts. Because I control my thoughts, I control my cravings.
• My cravings have no power—I do!
• I remain constantly aware of my thoughts.
• I am cleaning out the old, worn-out thoughts that no longer serve me.
• I halt my cravings by first hearing my thoughts.
• I listen to what I'm telling myself.
• I am a conscious eater.
• I can turn my non-constructive thoughts around in an instant!
• I focus on my strengths and positive attributes.
• I have a new set of beliefs that bring me the results I want.

Triggers
• When faced with a craving, I take a moment to HALT and find out what caused it.

• I identify my craving triggers and work to either eliminate them or deal with them in a healthy way.
• I no longer let the sight or smell of food lead me to overeat.

Limiting Beliefs
• I concentrate on positive thoughts.
• I have a new set of beliefs that works for me.
• What I tell myself is infinitely more important than what others tell me about myself.
• I work daily to clean out the false messages in my head.
• I can resist any food because food has no power—I do!
• I am perfectly happy skipping dessert.
• I no longer have the need to snack, but I give myself permission to eat between meals if it feels right.
• I can do anything I set my mind to.
• I am rooting out all the "can'ts" in my thoughts.
• I choose to take control of my life.
• I don't try; I *do!*
• I reword my thoughts to make them work for me.

Reprogramming Your Thoughts
• I have created a powerful arsenal of thoughts to conquer my cravings.
• I take the trouble to write down my affirmations because I'm worth it.
• I believe my affirmations and am seeing the results of using them.
• Whenever I call a HALT I find just the right affirmation to use at that moment.
• Using my affirmations is a daily priority.
• I am reprogramming my belief system to give me back my power.
• I realize I must work hard to change my beliefs, and my affirmations are the tools that are helping me do so.

Self -Esteem
• I am a good person, no matter what I eat.
• I am a good person, no matter how much I eat.
• I am strong and full of personal power!
• I love my body as it is and am making it more healthy every day.
• I am a beautiful person, inside and out!

- I accept all parts of my body and am thankful for my good health.
- I am worthy and loveable.
- I am good enough.
- I respect myself.
- I refuse to be controlled by society's idea of the ideal body.
- I am treating myself to an image make-over.
- I am the same loveable, worthy person, no matter what I weigh.
- People like me for who I am, not how I look.
- I accept the parts of me that I can't change.
- I receive compliments with pleasure and realize they are offered with sincerity.
- I approve of myself and need no one's approval but my own.
- I only apply labels to myself that serve my purposes.
- I am taking action to create positive labels for myself.
- I am redefining who I am, and I like that person!

Feelings
- I allow myself to feel all my emotions, good and bad.
- I am willing to face the emotions that have caused my cravings.
- I no longer stuff down my feelings with food.
- I don't do drugs, no matter how they're packaged!
- I enjoy food for what it is, but I no longer use it to numb myself.
- When I get a craving, I call a HALT, ask myself what I'm not allowing myself to feel, then find a healthy way to deal with it!
- I am a complete person, with positive and negative emotions.
- I feel my pain so that I can experience the joy of being whole.

Needs
- I am a loveable person with normal human needs.
- I feel no shame in looking for ways to meet my needs.
- Before I eat, I always ask myself if I am really hungry.
- When I get a craving, I HALT and ask myself what need my craving is trying to feed.
- I no longer use food as a substitute for love, nurturing, and attention.
- I no longer need my childhood eating habits. I am an adult now and find other ways of dealing with my needs.

Guilt, Shame, and Other Bugaboos
• If I eat something that isn't healthy, I make a conscious choice to eat better for the rest of the day.
• I am rooting out all the self-imposed "shoulds" and "shouldn'ts" that no longer serve me.
• I don't block my negative feelings. I deal with them.
• I look for solutions to my problems, then I take action to make them happen.
• I release my guilt by accepting my actions and taking responsibility for them.
• I channel my anger into a positive force that spurs me to action.
• I use my negative emotions as a sign that something in my life needs attention.
• Rather than blocking my negative feelings, I accept them, then allow them to wash through me.
• I dissolve my fears by facing them.
• I release my attention from worry, doubt, and fear.

Conscious Mental Dialoguing
• I deal with my emotions by having conscious mental dialogues with myself.
• I no longer struggle with craving voices. I ask myself objective questions and dig out the subconscious emotions that caused my craving in the first place.
• I refuse to be judgmental with myself. I am okay no matter what I do.

Visualization
• I prepare myself to succeed by visualizing my success.
• When I know I'm going to be faced with a craving trigger, I take a moment to HALT and visualize myself dealing with it in advance.
• I'm ready to face my challenges!

The Voice of Reason
• I look for support in handling my problems, rather than keeping them all to myself.
• By admitting my problems, I am better able to deal with them.

• I believe my intuition is a remarkable source of guidance that can help me conquer my cravings.
• I trust that my inner guide is always available to help me.
• I listen for the voice of my intuition and act on its advice.
• I am never alone. My inner guide is always with me.
• I differentiate between the different voices I hear and choose to listen to the wisest one, the voice of my intuition.
• I am filled with peace and energy because I am letting my inner guide direct my actions.
• Rather than remaining a victim, I ask my inner guide for the answers to my troubling questions.
• I recognize the advice from my intuition because I am in tune with my Self.

Let Your Inner Guide Handle It!
• I no longer try to control my eating through willpower. I let my inner guide do all the work.
• I trust my intuition to tell me when I should eat and how much I should eat.
• I listen to my body and eat when I am truly hungry.
• I relax my anxious thoughts about food.
• When I find myself struggling over whether or not to eat, I turn my struggle over to my inner guide.
• I maintain my ideal weight without effort.
• I give myself permission to eat, knowing my inner guide will let me know what's OK to eat and what isn't.
• I experience tremendous power by throwing away food that I really didn't want to eat in the first place.

Meditation
• I am my number one priority, and meditation is my way of taking care of myself.
• I reduce my stress and eliminate my cravings by taking time out of my busy day to meditate.

Be Your Own Best Friend
• I treat myself with the same kindness as I treat my friends.

• I am my best friend.
• I no longer look to food to bring me happiness—I create it from the inside out!
• I find creative alternatives for entertaining myself, rather than turning to food.
• If I get a craving, I call a HALT and take a good look at how I'm treating myself.
• I talk to myself kindly and patiently—just like I'd talk to a friend.

Loving Strategies

• I am no longer obsessed with the numbers on a scale. I monitor my weight in more healthy ways.
• Diets are gone from my life because I now deal with food in a healthy manner. I have replaced temporary solutions with long-term, positive lifestyle changes.
• I am making gradual changes in my eating habits that I can live with, without feeling deprived.
• I am free of dieting forever.
• I enjoy snacking because I make nutritious, enjoyable snacks a part of my regular eating habits.
• I eat foods that are healthy yet satisfying.
• I don't eat like that anymore!
• I enjoy my new eating habits.
• I love the new me!
• I have changed my attitude toward exercise and am making it part of my life.
• My body is capable of far more than I ever realized!
• I am a lean, mean, fighting machine!
• I love working out!
• I no longer make excuses for not exercising.
• I do my best and am perfectly happy not being perfect.

Revie wing the Process

• I am a conscious eater.
• I have broken free of the craving cycle.

Keeping a Journal

I enjoy writing in my journal and am achieving results much faster because of the effort I put into it.

• I review my journal regularly to learn from my behavior and remind myself of my successes.

Success and Setbacks

• I am a winner!

• I expect slipups, plan for them, and find ways to overcome them.

• If I eat more than I intended to, I ask myself why and figure out how to handle the situation better next time.

• I succeed at things because I know I can!

• I have the determination to succeed.

• I am motivated!

• I am focused on my goal of conquering my cravings and I will persevere until I succeed!

• I can handle anything life throws at me!

Goal-Setting

• My goal is to be free of cravings, and I am going for it!

• I have a plan of attack, and my victory is assured!

• I write down my goals and review them regularly. In this way I am ensuring my success!

• I love achieving my goals, one by one.

The Future

• I believe in me!

• I am building the life I've always dreamed of.

• I am living my life the way I've always wanted to!

• I am now the person I've always dreamed of being.

• I no longer have a problem with food.

• That was the old me.

• I have conquered my cravings!

• I am filled with enthusiasm and hope.

• I am unstoppable!

CPSIA information can be obtained
at www.ICGtesting.com
Printed in the USA
LVOW01s0007090317

526620LV00029B/934/P